W9-CEZ-343

Smart Heart

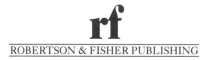

ROBERTSON & FISHER PUBLISHING

Written by: Dean J. Kereiakes, MD, FACC, and Douglas Wetherill, MS
Contributing Editors: Jenifer Jennings, PharmD, CDE; Paul Ribisl, PhD; Kristen Acra, RD, LD, CDE; Wayne M. Sotile, PhD; Rona Wharton, MEd, RD, LD; and Angela Ginty

Special thanks to George and Morfydd Wetherill for their layout and design contributions.

Cover Photographs: Photodisc Collection/Thinkstock/Digital Vision/Getty Images
Interior Photographs and Illustration: Getty Images. See credits.
Back Cover Photographs: Comstock/Mark Thorton/Mitch Hrdlicka/Getty Images

Robertson & Fisher Publishing Company
P.O. Box 8221
Cincinnati, OH 45208
513-373-2158

Printed in the United States of America

A catalog record for this book is available from the U.S. Library of Congress.

Recipes reprinted with permission from BETTY CROCKER HEALTHY HEART COOKBOOK: EVERYDAY MEALS, by the Betty Crocker Editors with Richard M. Bergenstal, MD, and Juli Hermanson, MPH, RD

Introduction

An important part of living with heart disease is understanding and monitoring your blood pressure, weight, and cholesterol values. You can learn to monitor changes in your body by writing down your weekly weight and blood pressure (if you have a home blood-pressure monitor). Your doctor might ask you to record your blood pressure every day, preferably at different times of day.

This journal also provides room for you to write down brief nutrition notes. One diet does not work for everyone with heart disease. It's a good idea to meet with a registered dietitian to review your lab results and lifestyle and to discuss your options. The diet you create together becomes a form of treatment — medical nutrition therapy — which is personalized just for you.

Controlling heart disease often requires you to monitor other aspects of your life as well. For example, if you have diabetes, you need to monitor your daily blood-sugar (blood-glucose) numbers. Monitoring your blood sugar helps your doctor evaluate your recommended treatment plan. Your doctor might ask you to monitor your blood sugar several times a day: before meals, at lunch, at dinner time, before bedtime, and before/after exercising.

Your doctor has probably recommended a light exercise program. If you are just starting to exercise, check with your doctor before you begin your program. He or she will be aware of the many factors that may need to be considered limitations regarding your exercise program.

To begin, try to commit yourself to exercise at least 5 to 10 minutes daily for the first few weeks. This will help you establish a more consistent exercise routine. Use this journal to note your exercise days and duration. This allows you to track your progress and reinforces the changes you are making.

You may also use the space in your journal to keep up with doctor appointments, sick days, and questions that you want to remember to ask your doctor, dietitian, or certified diabetes educator.

Heart disease is a complex condition that requires consistent attention, but monitoring your daily habits can have its rewards. You may not be able to completely reverse your condition, but you can take simple steps to maintain and enjoy your daily activities.

Treatment Disclaimer

This journal is for educational purposes, not for use in the treatment of medical conditions. It is based on skilled medical opinion as of the date of publication. However, medical science advances and changes rapidly. Furthermore, diagnosis and treatment are often complex and involve more than one disease process or medical issue to determine proper care. If you believe you may have a medical condition described in the journal, consult your doctor.

Journal Topics

Journal

Getting Started

Heart disease is a complex condition that requires consistent attention — but your efforts to improve your overall health can pay big dividends and possibly reduce the risk of another heart event.

Managing your heart health means working closely with your doctor and heart-care team. More than likely, your doctor has prescribed several medications, diet modification, and an exercise routine to help improve your cardiac condition. Your doctor may ask you to monitor your blood pressure and weight throughout the week to ensure the lifestyle changes are meeting your needs.

However, you must remember that the most important person in your healthcare team is YOU. Managing heart disease requires commitment to make the necessary changes – whether it is remembering to take your medication, modifying the portions in your diet, or sticking with an exercise routine. Your healthcare team is there to help you . . . and they want you to succeed.

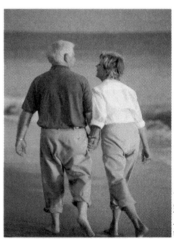

If your doctor approves, start a simple exercise program — like walking or swimming.

Do not let what you cannot do interfere with what you can do.
—John Wooden

Notes

MONDAY

Minutes of exercise _____
Weight _____
Blood pressure _____

TUESDAY

Minutes of exercise _____
Weight _____
Blood pressure _____

WEDNESDAY

Minutes of exercise _____
Weight _____
Blood pressure _____

THURSDAY

Minutes of exercise _____
Weight _____
Blood pressure _____

FRIDAY

Minutes of exercise _____
Weight _____
Blood pressure _____

SATURDAY

Minutes of exercise _____
Weight _____
Blood pressure _____

SUNDAY

Minutes of exercise _____
Weight _____
Blood pressure _____

Things to do for next week:

Check next week's supply of:
- ○ blood pressure medication
- ○ cholesterol medication
- ○ aspirin
- ○ vitamins
- ○ diabetes medication
- ○ lancets
- ○ glucose test strips

Plum-Glazed Turkey Tenderloins

PREP: 10 min MARINATE: 30 min GRILL: 30 min

Ingredients
1/4 cup dry sherry or chicken broth
1/4 teaspoon pepper
2 tablespoons olive or canola oil
1 1/2 teaspoons garlic salt
1 medium onion, finely chopped (1/2 cup)
1 cup plum jam or any fruit jam
2 teaspoons chopped fresh or 1/2 teaspoon dried rosemary leaves, crumbled
1 1/2 pounds turkey breast tenderloins (about 3 tenderloins)

1   Mix all ingredients except turkey in medium bowl. Place turkey in shallow glass or plastic dish or heavy-duty resealable plastic food-storage bag. Pour half of the plum mixture over turkey; turn turkey to coat. Reserve remaining half of plum mixture. Cover dish or seal bag and refrigerate 30 minutes, turning once.

2   If using charcoal grill, place drip pan directly under grilling area, and arrange coals around edge of firebox. Heat coals or gas grill for indirect heat.

3   Remove turkey from marinade; reserve marinade for basting. Cover and grill turkey over drip pan or over unheated side of gas grill and 4 to 6 inches from medium-high heat 25 to 30 minutes, turning and brushing with reserved basting marinade occasionally, until juice of turkey is no longer pink when centers of thickest pieces are cut. Discard any remaining basting marinade.

4   Heat reserved plum mixture. Serve with sliced turkey.

2 Carbohydrate Choices

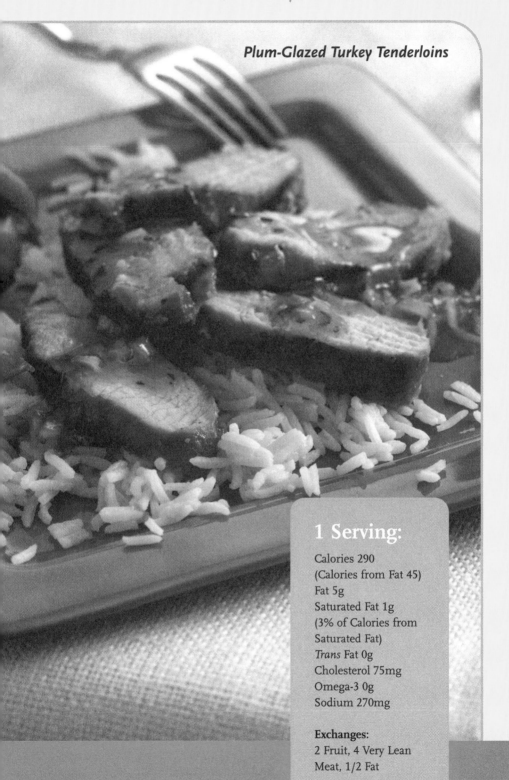

Plum-Glazed Turkey Tenderloins

1 Serving:

Calories 290
(Calories from Fat 45)
Fat 5g
Saturated Fat 1g
(3% of Calories from
Saturated Fat)
Trans Fat 0g
Cholesterol 75mg
Omega-3 0g
Sodium 270mg

Exchanges:
2 Fruit, 4 Very Lean
Meat, 1/2 Fat

Your Healthcare Team

Improving your cardiac condition is a team effort. Your healthcare team will determine the frequency of your visits. As a guideline, every year, you could see the members of your healthcare team according to the following schedule:

- Family doctor   3 times
- Cardiologist   2 times
- Registered dietitian   1 time

If you have both cardiovascular disease and diabetes, it is important for you to schedule, on average, regular appointments with other specialists (endocrinologist, ophthalmologist, certified diabetes educator). Here is the recommended schedule for people who also have diabetes:

- Endocrinologist   2 times
- Dentist   2 times
- Ophthalmologist   1 time
- Podiatrist   1 time
- Certified diabetes educator   1 time

See your doctors on a regular schedule.

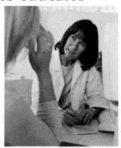

Digital Vision/Getty Images

Notes

MONDAY

Minutes of exercise _____
Weight _____
Blood pressure _____

TUESDAY

Minutes of exercise _____
Weight _____
Blood pressure _____

WEDNESDAY

Minutes of exercise _____
Weight _____
Blood pressure _____

THURSDAY

Minutes of exercise _____
Weight _____
Blood pressure _____

FRIDAY

Minutes of exercise _____
Weight _____
Blood pressure _____

SATURDAY

Minutes of exercise _____
Weight _____
Blood pressure _____

SUNDAY

Minutes of exercise _____
Weight _____
Blood pressure _____

Things to do for next week:

Check next week's supply of:
- ○ blood pressure medication
- ○ cholesterol medication
- ○ aspirin
- ○ vitamins
- ○ diabetes medication
- ○ lancets
- ○ glucose test strips

Grilled Salmon with Hazelnut Butter

PREP: 10 min GRILL: 10 min
4 servings

Ingredients
Hazelnut Butter (below)
1 pound salmon, trout or other medium-firm fish fillets
1/2 teaspoon salt
1/8 teaspoon pepper

1   Brush grill rack with canola or soybean oil. Heat coals or gas
    grill for direct heat. Make Hazelnut Butter; set aside.

2   If fish fillets are large, cut into 4 serving pieces. Sprinkle both
    sides of fish with salt and pepper.

3   Cover and grill fish 4 to 6 inches from medium heat
    4 minutes. Turn; spread about 1 tablespoon hazelnut butter
    over each fillet. Cover and grill 4 to 6 minutes longer or until
    fish flakes easily with fork.

Hazelnut Butter
2 tablespoons finely chopped hazelnuts
1 tablespoon chopped fresh parsley
2 tablespoons butter, softened
1 teaspoon lemon juice

Spread nuts in shallow
microwavable bowl or pie plate.
Microwave uncovered on High
30 seconds to 1 minute, stirring
once or twice, until light brown;
cool. Mix hazelnuts and remaining
ingredients in small bowl.

1 Serving:

Calories 230
(Calories from Fat 125)
Fat 14g
Saturated Fat 6g
(22% of Calories from
Saturated Fat)
Trans Fat 0g
Cholesterol 90mg
Omega-3 0g
Sodium 400mg

Exchanges:
3 1/2 Lean Meat, 1 Fat

0 Carbohydrate Choices

Asian Steak Salad

PREP: 15 min COOK: 5 min
4 servings

Ingredients
1 pound cut-up beef for stir-fry
1 package (3 ounces) Oriental-flavor ramen noodle soup
  mix
1/2 cup Asian marinade and dressing
1 bag (10 ounces) romaine and leaf lettuce mix
1 cup fresh snow (Chinese) pea pods
1/2 cup matchstick-cut carrots (from 10-ounce bag)
1 can (11 ounces) mandarin orange segments, drained

1 Serving:

Calories 185
(Calories from Fat 25)
Fat 3g
Saturated Fat 1g
(5% of Calories from
Saturated Fat)
Trans Fat 0g
Cholesterol 40mg
Omega-3 0g
Sodium 570mg

Exchanges:
2 Very Lean Meat

1   Spray 12-inch nonstick skillet with cooking
    spray; heat over medium-high heat. Place beef
    in skillet; sprinkle with 1 teaspoon seasoning mix from soup
    mix. (Discard remaining seasoning mix.) Cook beef 4 to
    5 minutes, stirring occasionally, until brown. Stir in
    1 tablespoon of the dressing.

2   Break block of noodles from soup mix into small pieces.
    Mix noodles, lettuce, pea pods, carrots and orange segments
    in large bowl. Add remaining dressing; toss until well coated.
    Divide mixture among individual serving plates. Top with
    beef strips.

3 Carbohydrate Choices

Going to the Doctor

Be prepared for every visit to your doctor, registered dietitian, and other members of your healthcare team. For each visit, you should take:

- A current/updated list of your medical conditions — including any changes since your last visit
- A list of all your medications and doses (include aspirin, vitamins, and herbs)
- A list of questions you have — and a pen and your journal to record the answers

Be on time. Call 24 hours in advance if you cannot keep an appointment.

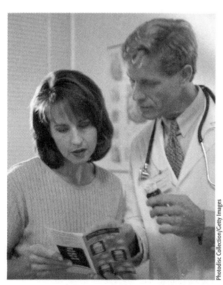

Talk to your doctor or pharmacist about your medications.

Photodisc Collection/Getty Images

People want to know how much you care before they care about how much you know.
—James F. Hind

Notes

MONDAY

Minutes of exercise _____
Weight _____
Blood pressure _____

TUESDAY

Minutes of exercise _____
Weight _____
Blood pressure _____

WEDNESDAY

Minutes of exercise _____
Weight _____
Blood pressure _____

THURSDAY

Minutes of exercise _____
Weight _____
Blood pressure _____

FRIDAY

Minutes of exercise _____
Weight _____
Blood pressure _____

SATURDAY

Minutes of exercise _____
Weight _____
Blood pressure _____

SUNDAY

Minutes of exercise _____
Weight _____
Blood pressure _____

Things to do for next week:

Check next week's supply of:
- ○ blood pressure medication
- ○ cholesterol medication
- ○ aspirin
- ○ vitamins
- ○ diabetes medication
- ○ lancets
- ○ glucose test strips

Grilled Halibut with Tomato-Avocado Salsa

PREP: 20 min MARINATE: 30 min GRILL: 15 min

Ingredients
2 tablespoons canola or soybean oil
2 tablespoons lemon or lime juice
1/4 teaspoon salt
1/4 teaspoon ground cumin
1 clove garlic, finely chopped
1 1/2 pounds halibut, tuna or
  swordfish steaks, 3/4 to 1 inch thick
1/8 teaspoon ground red pepper (cayenne)

Tomato-Avocado Salsa
3 medium tomatoes, chopped
  (1 1/2 cups)
1 medium avocado, pitted, peeled
  and coarsely chopped
1 small jalapeño chili, seeded and
  finely chopped
1/4 cup chopped fresh cilantro
2 teaspoons lemon or lime juice
Mix all ingredients in medium
bowl.

1 If fish steaks are large, cut into 6 serving pieces. Mix remaining
   ingredients except Tomato-Avocado Salsa in shallow glass or
   plastic dish. Add fish; turn to coat with marinade. Cover and
   refrigerate at least 30 minutes but no longer than 2 hours.

2 Heat coals or gas grill for direct heat. Remove fish from
   marinade; reserve marinade. Cover and grill fish 4 to 5 inches
   from medium heat 10 to 15 minutes, brushing 2 or
   3 times with marinade and
   turning once, until fish flakes
   easily with fork. Discard any
   remaining marinade.

3 While fish is grilling, make
   Tomato-Avocado Salsa. Serve
   fish with salsa.

1 Serving:

Calories 205
(Calories from Fat 90)
Fat 10g
Saturated Fat 1g
(3% of Calories from
Saturated Fat)
Trans Fat 0g
Cholesterol 60mg
Omega-3 1g
Sodium 170mg

Exchanges:
1 Vegetable, 3 Lean Meat

0.5 Carbohydrate Choices

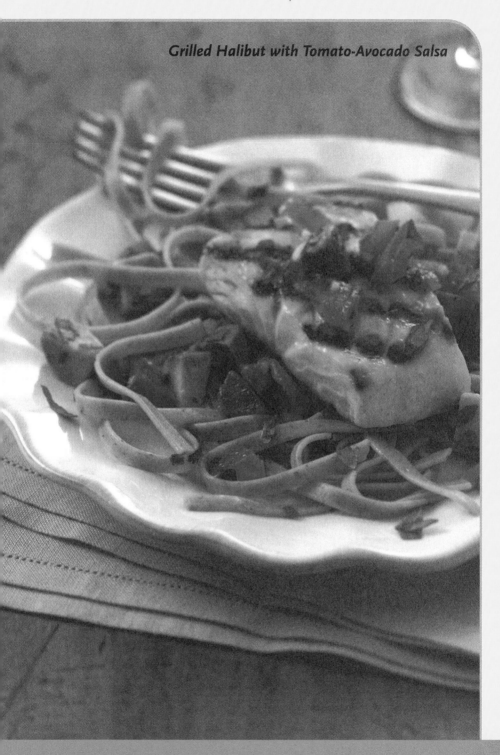

Grilled Halibut with Tomato-Avocado Salsa

Quick Breakfast Ideas

Eating breakfast is very important for everyone. Finding the time for breakfast can be challenging. To avoid skipping this very important meal, try some of these quick-and-easy breakfast ideas:

- 1 cup sugar-free yogurt with 3/4 cup fresh berries topped with 1 tablespoon granola
- 1 whole wheat bagel with 1 tablespoon natural peanut butter or low-fat margarine and 1 to 2 teaspoons low-sugar jelly
- 1 hard-boiled egg, 1 piece of toast, and 1/2 cup juice
- Unsweetened cold cereal with 1% or skim milk
- Frozen waffles topped with berries
- Instant oatmeal
- Smoothie made from sugar-free yogurt and your favorite fresh or frozen berries and a couple of ice cubes

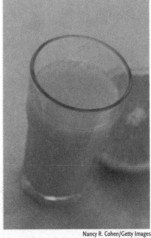

Nancy R. Cohen/Getty Images

Try to include a glass of juice, like orange juice, in your breakfast meal plan.

You will make mistakes; but as long as you are generous and true, and also fierce, you cannot hurt the world or even seriously distress her. —Winston Churchill

MONDAY

Minutes of exercise _____
Weight _____
Blood pressure _____

TUESDAY

Minutes of exercise _____
Weight _____
Blood pressure _____

WEDNESDAY

Minutes of exercise _____
Weight _____
Blood pressure _____

THURSDAY

Minutes of exercise _____
Weight _____
Blood pressure _____

FRIDAY

Minutes of exercise _____
Weight _____
Blood pressure _____

SATURDAY

Minutes of exercise _____
Weight _____
Blood pressure _____

SUNDAY

Minutes of exercise _____
Weight _____
Blood pressure _____

Things to do for next week:

Check next week's supply of:
- ○ vitamins
- ○ blood pressure medication
- ○ diabetes medication
- ○ cholesterol medication
- ○ lancets
- ○ aspirin
- ○ glucose test strips

Spinach Quesadillas with Feta Cheese

PREP: 15 min   COOK: 2 min
4 servings

Ingredients
4 fat-free flour tortillas (8 inches in diameter)
1/4 cup soft reduced-fat cream cheese with roasted garlic
2 cups frozen chopped spinach, thawed and squeezed to drain
1 tablespoon finely chopped red onion
1/4 cup crumbled feta cheese (1 ounce)
16 cherry tomatoes
2 tablespoons fat-free sour cream
1/4 cup sliced ripe olives

1   Spread 2 tortillas with cream cheese. Layer spinach, onion and feta cheese over cream cheese. Top with remaining 2 tortillas; press lightly.

2   Spray 12-inch nonstick skillet with cooking spray; heat over medium heat. Cook each quesadilla in skillet 2 to 3 minutes on each side or until light golden brown.

3   Cut each quesadilla into 8 wedges. Cut cherry tomatoes in half; top with sour cream, tomato halves and olives. Secure with toothpicks. Serve warm.

1 Serving:

Calories 230
(Calories from Fat 125)
Fat 14g
Saturated Fat 6g
(22% of Calories from
Saturated Fat)
Trans Fat 0g
Cholesterol 90mg
Omega-3 0g
Sodium 400mg

0.5 Carbohydrate Choices

Exchanges:
3 1/2 Lean Meat, 1 Fat

French Toast with Gingered Applesauce

PREP: 15 min COOK: 2 min
4 servings

Ingredients
1/2 to 1 teaspoon grated gingerroot or 1/8 teaspoon ground ginger
1/2 cup unsweetened applesauce
1/4 cup sugar-free maple-flavored syrup
3/4 cup fat-free cholesterol-free egg product or 2 eggs plus 1 egg white
3/4 cup fat-free (skim) milk
1 teaspoon vanilla
1/4 teaspoon salt
8 slices whole-wheat sandwich bread or 1-inch-thick slices French bread

1 Mix gingerroot, applesauce and syrup in small microwavable bowl. Microwave uncovered on Medium (50%) about 1 minute or until very warm; set aside.

2 Beat egg product, milk, vanilla and salt in small bowl with fork or wire whisk until well mixed; pour into shallow bowl.

3 Spray griddle or 10-inch skillet with cooking spray; heat griddle to 375° or heat skillet over medium heat. Dip bread into egg mixture, coating both sides; place in skillet. Cook about 2 minutes on each side or until golden brown. Serve with applesauce mixture.

1 Serving:

Calories 205
(Calories from Fat 25)
Fat 3g
Saturated Fat 1g
(2% of Calories from Saturated Fat)
Trans Fat 0g
Cholesterol 0mg
Omega-3 0g
Sodium 590mg

Exchanges:
2 Starch, 1/2 Fruit,
1/2 Very Lean Meat

2.5 Carbohydrate Choices

Preparing to Exercise

If you have had a heart attack, bypass surgery or angioplasty, your cardiologist will likely ask you to have a treadmill test prior to beginning an exercise program. After the test, the doctor will be able to determine whether you have any exercise limitations or special considerations. Ask your doctor for recommendations and goals for your program.

If you also have diabetes, you should monitor your blood sugar and check your feet prior to each exercise session.

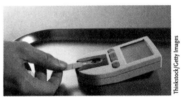

Check your blood sugar before and after you exercise.

If your blood sugar is too high (more than 240 mg/dL), test your urine for ketones with a special test strip. If ketones are present in your urine, you should not exercise. Call your doctor.

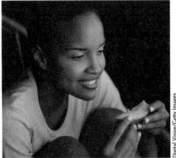

If your blood sugar is low, eat a light snack before you exercise.

If your blood sugar is too low (less than 100 mg/dL), you probably do not have enough energy to exercise safely. You should eat a light snack with 15 grams of carbohydrates — such as a piece of fruit or several graham crackers — and then exercise.

There is a kind of victory in good work, no matter how humble.
—Jack Kemp

Notes

MONDAY

Minutes of exercise _____
Weight _____
Blood pressure _____

TUESDAY

Minutes of exercise _____
Weight _____
Blood pressure _____

WEDNESDAY

Minutes of exercise _____
Weight _____
Blood pressure _____

THURSDAY

Minutes of exercise _____
Weight _____
Blood pressure _____

FRIDAY

Minutes of exercise _____
Weight _____
Blood pressure _____

SATURDAY

Minutes of exercise _____
Weight _____
Blood pressure _____

SUNDAY

Minutes of exercise _____
Weight _____
Blood pressure _____

Things to do for next week:

Check next week's supply of:
- ○ blood pressure medication
- ○ cholesterol medication
- ○ aspirin
- ○ vitamins
- ○ diabetes medication
- ○ lancets
- ○ glucose test strips

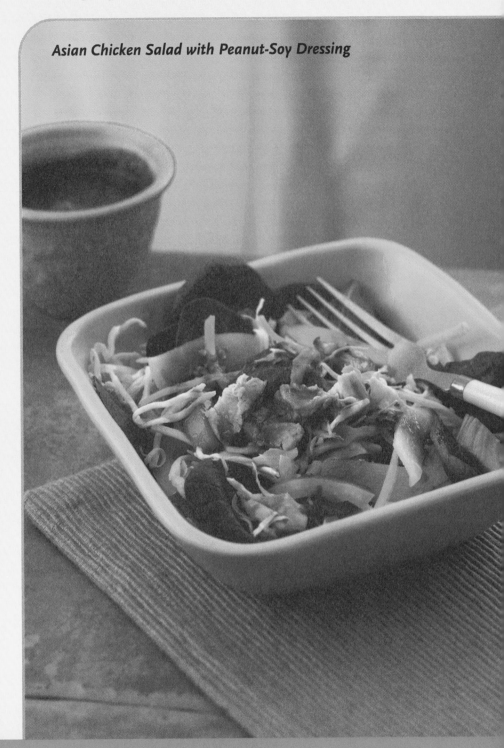

Asian Chicken Salad with Peanut-Soy Dressing

Asian Chicken Salad with Peanut-Soy Dressing

PREP: 15 min
6 servings

Ingredients
6 cups coleslaw mix (from 16-ounce bag)
3 cups washed fresh spinach leaves (from 10-ounce bag)
3 cups cut-up cooked chicken
1 medium bell pepper, cut into bite-size strips
1 can (8 ounces) bamboo shoots, rinsed and drained

Make Peanut-Soy Dressing. Toss remaining ingredients in large bowl; drizzle with dressing.

Peanut-Soy Dressing
3 tablespoons reduced-sodium soy sauce
3 tablespoons cider vinegar
2 tablespoons honey
1 tablespoon creamy peanut butter
1/2 teaspoon crushed red pepper
1/2 teaspoon grated gingerroot

Beat all ingredients in small bowl with wire whisk until blended.

1 Serving:

Calories 210
(Calories from Fat 65)
Fat 7g
Saturated Fat 2g
(8% of Calories from
Saturated Fat)
Trans Fat 0g
Cholesterol 60mg
Omega-3 0g
Sodium 360mg

Exchanges:
3 Vegetable,
2 1/2 Lean Meat

3 Carbohydrate Choices

You Are in Control

Regular exercise and proper diet will help maintain your physical health. Annual physical examinations by your doctor can screen for illness and help treat or cure any medical illnesses you may have.

Strong spiritual and mental health will help decrease stress in your life. Stress causes your brain to release signals to the body through the nerves, triggering various responses. Undue stress can lead to anxiety, depression, and tension. Try meditation, deep-breathing exercises, listening to music, or even going for a walk to reduce stress.

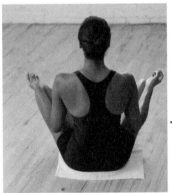

Try meditation or relaxation as a means for reducing stress.

Ryan McVay/Getty Images

Notes

MONDAY

Minutes of exercise _____
Weight _____
Blood pressure _____

TUESDAY

Minutes of exercise _____
Weight _____
Blood pressure _____

WEDNESDAY

Minutes of exercise _____
Weight _____
Blood pressure _____

THURSDAY

Minutes of exercise _____
Weight _____
Blood pressure _____

FRIDAY

Minutes of exercise _____
Weight _____
Blood pressure _____

SATURDAY

Minutes of exercise _____
Weight _____
Blood pressure _____

SUNDAY

Minutes of exercise _____
Weight _____
Blood pressure _____

Things to do for next week:

Check next week's supply of:
- ○ blood pressure medication
- ○ cholesterol medication
- ○ aspirin
- ○ vitamins
- ○ diabetes medication
- ○ lancets
- ○ glucose test strips

Berry-Banana Smoothie

PREP: 10 min
2 servings (about 1 cup each)

Ingredients
1 cup vanilla, plain, strawberry or raspberry fat-free yogurt
1/2 cup Cheerios® or another round oat cereal
2 tablespoons ground flaxseed or flaxseed meal
1/2 cup fresh strawberry halves or raspberries, or frozen whole strawberries
1/2 cup fat-free (skim) milk
1 to 2 tablespoons sugar
1/2 banana

1   Place all ingredients in blender. Cover and blend on high speed 10 seconds; stop blender to scrape sides. Cover and blend about 20 seconds longer or until smooth.

2   Pour mixture into glasses. Serve immediately.

1 Serving:

Calories 245
(Calories from Fat 35)
Fat 4g
Saturated Fat 1g
(2% of Calories from
Saturated Fat)
Trans Fat 0g
Cholesterol 5mg
Omega-3 0g
Sodium 150mg

Exchanges:
2 Fruit, 1 Milk, 1 Fat

3 Carbohydrate Choices

Roasted Red Pepper Bruschetta

PREP: 10 min BAKE: 8 min
12 appetizers

Ingredients
4 slices hard-crusted Italian or French bread, 1/2 inch thick
1 jar (7 ounces) roasted red bell peppers, drained and cut into 1/2-inch strips
1 or 2 medium cloves garlic, finely chopped
2 tablespoons chopped fresh parsley or 1 teaspoon parsley flakes
2 tablespoons shredded Parmesan cheese
1 tablespoon olive, canola or soybean oil
1/4 teaspoon salt
1/4 teaspoon pepper
1 tablespoon capers, drained

1   Heat oven to 450°. Place bread on ungreased cookie sheet. Mix remaining ingredients except capers in small bowl. Spoon onto bread, spreading evenly.

2   Bake 6 to 8 minutes or until edges of bread are golden brown. Cut each slice lengthwise into thirds. Sprinkle with capers.

1 Appetizer:

Calories 40
(Calories from Fat 20)
Fat 2g
Saturated Fat 0g
(8% of Calories from
Saturated Fat)
Trans Fat 0g
Cholesterol 0mg
Omega-3 0g
Sodium 125mg

Exchanges:
1/2 Starch

0 Carbohydrate Choices

Exercise 101

For the beginner, the simplest exercise is walking. Always check with your doctor about possible exercise limitations.

Start with a 5- to 10-minute walk each day and increase your duration by 1 to 2 minutes per week, whichever feels comfortable. Work up to a 30-minute walk every day over the next 6 months.

Start slowly with consistency and patience, and do something every day to gradually build up your exercise capacity. Make a long-term commitment and stick to it.

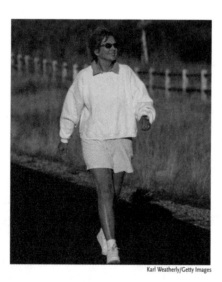

Karl Weatherly/Getty Images

If your schedule permits, try to walk on a daily basis.

It's better to be a lion for a day than a sheep all your life.
—Sister Kenny

Notes

MONDAY

Minutes of exercise _____
Weight _____
Blood pressure _____

TUESDAY

Minutes of exercise _____
Weight _____
Blood pressure _____

WEDNESDAY

Minutes of exercise _____
Weight _____
Blood pressure _____

THURSDAY

Minutes of exercise _____
Weight _____
Blood pressure _____

FRIDAY

Minutes of exercise _____
Weight _____
Blood pressure _____

SATURDAY

Minutes of exercise _____
Weight _____
Blood pressure _____

SUNDAY

Minutes of exercise _____
Weight _____
Blood pressure _____

Things to do for next week:

Check next week's supply of:
- ○ blood pressure medication
- ○ cholesterol medication
- ○ aspirin
- ○ vitamins
- ○ diabetes medication
- ○ lancets
- ○ glucose test strips

Baked Apple Oatmeal

PREP: 15 min BAKE: 45 min
8 servings

Ingredients
2 2/3 cups old-fashioned oats
1/2 cup raisins
1/3 cup packed brown sugar
1 teaspoon ground cinnamon
1/4 teaspoon salt
4 cups fat-free (skim) milk
2 medium apples or pears, chopped (2 cups)
1/2 cup chopped walnuts
Additional fat-free (skim) milk, if desired

1 Heat oven to 350°. Mix oats, raisins, brown sugar, cinnamon, salt and 4 cups milk and the apples in 2-quart casserole.

2 Bake uncovered 40 to 45 minutes or until most liquid is absorbed. Sprinkle walnuts over top. Serve with additional milk.

1 Serving:

Calories 270
(Calories from Fat 65)
Fat 7g
Saturated Fat 1g
(3% of Calories from
Saturated Fat)
Trans Fat 0g
Cholesterol 0mg
Omega-3 1g
Sodium 140mg

Exchanges:
1 Starch, 1 Fruit,
1 Milk, 1 Fat

2.5 Carbohydrate Choices

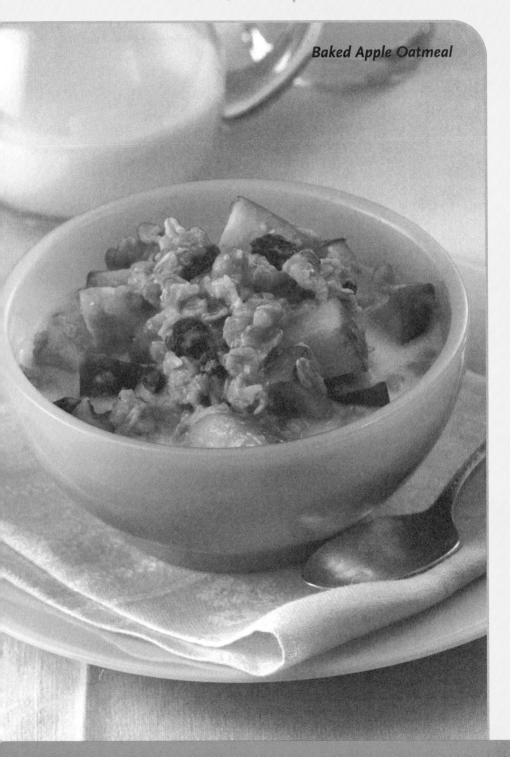

Baked Apple Oatmeal

Depression

Depression is a medical condition that can affect you in many ways.

Mood
- Sad
- Loss of joy
- Grouchy
- Angry

Thinking
- Gloomy outlook
- Poor concentration
- Memory problems

Behavior
- Difficulty getting work or chores done
- Avoid dealing with other people

Body Functions
- Poor sleep
- Weight loss or gain
- Low sex drive
- Low energy

If you have any of these symptoms for more than 3 weeks, ask your doctor if counseling or medication might help. Each day, whether you feel like it or not, follow through with some of your duties (this will give you a sense of achievement) and do at least one thing that would normally bring you pleasure. If you begin to feel hopeless or think of hurting yourself, get help now!

All things are possible until they are proved impossible — and even the impossible may only be so as of now.
—Pearl S. Buck

Notes

MONDAY

Minutes of exercise _____
Weight _____
Blood pressure _____

TUESDAY

Minutes of exercise _____
Weight _____
Blood pressure _____

WEDNESDAY

Minutes of exercise _____
Weight _____
Blood pressure _____

THURSDAY

Minutes of exercise _____
Weight _____
Blood pressure _____

FRIDAY

Minutes of exercise _____
Weight _____
Blood pressure _____

SATURDAY

Minutes of exercise _____
Weight _____
Blood pressure _____

SUNDAY

Minutes of exercise _____
Weight _____
Blood pressure _____

Things to do for next week:

Check next week's supply of:
○ blood pressure medication
○ cholesterol medication
○ aspirin
○ vitamins
○ diabetes medication
○ lancets
○ glucose test strips

Potato-Crusted Salmon

PREP: 10 min COOK: 6 min
4 servings

Ingredients
1 egg white
2 tablespoons water
1/3 cup plain mashed potato mix (dry)
2 teaspoons cornstarch
1 teaspoon paprika
1 teaspoon lemon pepper seasoning salt
1 tablespoon canola or soybean oil
1 pound salmon, arctic char or other medium-firm fish fillets,
  about 3/4 inch thick

1   Remove and discard skin from fish. Cut fish into 4 serving
    pieces. Beat egg white and water slightly with fork in shallow
    dish.

2   Mix potato mix, cornstarch, paprika and lemon pepper in
    another shallow dish. Dip just the top sides of fish into egg
    white mixture, then press into potato mixture.

3   Spray 12-inch nonstick skillet with
    cooking spray. Heat oil in skillet
    over high heat. Cook fish, potato
    sides down, in oil 3 minutes.
    Carefully turn fish, using wide
    slotted spatula. Reduce heat to
    medium. Cook about 3 minutes
    longer or until fish flakes easily
    with fork.

1 Serving:

Calories 190
(Calories from Fat 80)
Fat 9g
Saturated Fat 2g
(9% of Calories from
Saturated Fat)
Trans Fat 0g
Cholesterol 65mg
Omega-3 2g
Sodium 420mg

Exchanges:
1/2 Other Carbohydrates,
3 Lean Meat

0.5 Carbohydrate Choices

Spicy Chicken Drumsticks

PREP: 20 min BAKE: 45 min
5 servings

Ingredients
2 pounds chicken drumsticks
1/3 cup all-purpose flour
1/3 cup yellow whole-grain cornmeal
1/2 teaspoon ground cumin
1/2 teaspoon chili powder
1/4 teaspoon salt
1/3 cup buttermilk
1/4 teaspoon red pepper sauce
Cooking spray

1 Serving:

Calories 185
(Calories from Fat 35)
Fat 4g
Saturated Fat 1g
(6% of Calories from
Saturated Fat)
Trans Fat 0g
Cholesterol 85mg
Omega-3 0g
Sodium 200mg

Exchanges:
1 Starch, 3 Very Lean Meat

1 Heat oven to 400°. Spray rectangular pan,
   13 x 9 x 2 inches, with cooking spray. Remove
   skin and fat from chicken.

2 Mix flour, cornmeal, cumin, chili powder and salt in
   heavy-duty resealable plastic food-storage bag. Mix
   buttermilk and pepper sauce in medium bowl. Dip chicken
   into buttermilk mixture, then place in bag. Seal bag and
   shake until evenly coated. Place chicken in pan; spray chicken
   lightly with cooking spray.

3 Bake uncovered 40 to 45 minutes or until juice of chicken is
   no longer pink when centers of thickest pieces are cut.

1 Carbohydrate Choice

Weight-Loss Tips

If you are overweight, losing a few pounds, even 5% to 10% of your body weight, will help you to control your blood-sugar levels. Weight loss will also help you control your cholesterol and blood pressure. The recommended rate of weight loss is 1 to 2 pounds per week. Try some of these tips to get on the road to weight loss:

- Eat a wide variety of foods from all food groups.
- Avoid skipping meals. It may be best to eat small, frequent meals.
- Control portion sizes. It may be helpful to measure and weigh foods for a better understanding of portion sizes.
- Eat slowly.
- Keep a food journal. (See page 110.)
- Incorporate aerobic activity into your lifestyle. Remember to consult with your physician before beginning an exercise program.
- Consult with a registered dietitian for an individualized weight-loss plan.

Weigh yourself one time per week on the same day at approximately the same time.

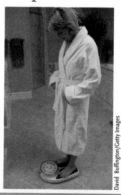

David Buffington/Getty Images

How we spend our days is, of course, how we spend our lives.
—Annie Dillard

Notes

MONDAY

Minutes of exercise _____
Weight _____
Blood pressure _____

TUESDAY

Minutes of exercise _____
Weight _____
Blood pressure _____

WEDNESDAY

Minutes of exercise _____
Weight _____
Blood pressure _____

THURSDAY

Minutes of exercise _____
Weight _____
Blood pressure _____

FRIDAY

Minutes of exercise _____
Weight _____
Blood pressure _____

SATURDAY

Minutes of exercise _____
Weight _____
Blood pressure _____

SUNDAY

Minutes of exercise _____
Weight _____
Blood pressure _____

Things to do for next week:

Check next week's supply of:
○ blood pressure medication
○ cholesterol medication
○ aspirin
○ vitamins
○ diabetes medication
○ lancets
○ glucose test strips

Dijon Chicken Smothered in Mushrooms

PREP: 10 min COOK: 12 min
4 servings

Ingredients
4 boneless skinless chicken breast halves (about 1 pound) or 1-pound pork
  tenderloin
1/4 cup all-purpose flour
1/2 teaspoon salt
1/4 teaspoon pepper
2 tablespoons olive or canola oil
1/2 cup roasted garlic-seasoned chicken broth (from 14-ounce can)
1 1/2 tablespoons Dijon mustard
1 jar (4 1/2 ounces) sliced mushrooms, drained
Chopped fresh thyme, if desired

1   If using pork, cut into 1-inch-thick slices. Place chicken (or pork) between 2 sheets of plastic wrap or waxed paper. Flatten chicken to 1/4-inch thickness with meat mallet or rolling pin. Mix flour, salt and pepper in shallow dish.

2   Heat oil in 12-inch nonstick skillet over medium-high heat. Coat both sides of chicken with flour mixture. Cook chicken in hot oil 6 to 8 minutes, turning once, until chicken is no longer pink in center (pork is no longer pink and meat thermometer inserted in center reads 160°). Remove chicken to serving plate; cover to keep warm.

3   Stir broth into skillet. Heat to boiling over medium-high heat. Stir in mustard and mushrooms. Cook 2 to 3 minutes, stirring frequently, until slightly thickened. Spoon sauce over chicken. Sprinkle with thyme.

0.5 Carbohydrate Choices

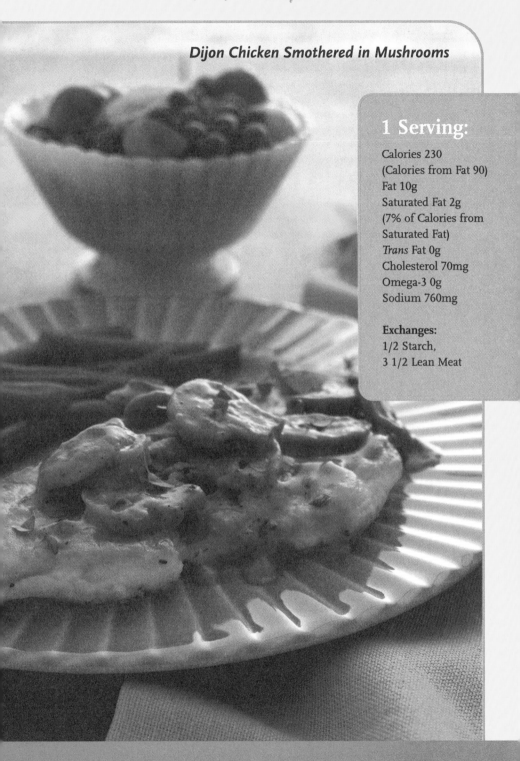

Dijon Chicken Smothered in Mushrooms

1 Serving:

Calories 230
(Calories from Fat 90)
Fat 10g
Saturated Fat 2g
(7% of Calories from
Saturated Fat)
Trans Fat 0g
Cholesterol 70mg
Omega-3 0g
Sodium 760mg

Exchanges:
1/2 Starch,
3 1/2 Lean Meat

Trans Fatty Acids

Trans fatty acids are a type of fatty acid formed during the process of hydrogenation of vegetable oils. They are found in vegetable shortening, some margarines, fried foods, and commercially baked goods, such as crackers, cookies, and cakes, and help to prolong the shelf life of certain foods. Trans fats are similar to saturated fats in that they can cause an increase in LDL-cholesterol levels and a decrease in HDL-cholesterol levels.

Look for the words "hydrogenated" or "partially hydrogenated" on the ingredient list of a food label to discover if that food contains high amounts of trans fatty acids.

It is best to use a liquid oil, preferably olive or canola oil, and to avoid trans fats.

Notes

MONDAY

Minutes of exercise _____
Weight _____
Blood pressure _____

TUESDAY

Minutes of exercise _____
Weight _____
Blood pressure _____

WEDNESDAY

Minutes of exercise _____
Weight _____
Blood pressure _____

THURSDAY

Minutes of exercise _____
Weight _____
Blood pressure _____

FRIDAY

Minutes of exercise _____
Weight _____
Blood pressure _____

SATURDAY

Minutes of exercise _____
Weight _____
Blood pressure _____

SUNDAY

Minutes of exercise _____
Weight _____
Blood pressure _____

Things to do for next week:

Check next week's supply of:

- ○ blood pressure medication
- ○ cholesterol medication
- ○ aspirin
- ○ vitamins
- ○ diabetes medication
- ○ lancets
- ○ glucose test strips

Loaded Potatoes

PREP: 12 min COOK: 4 min STAND: 4 min
4 servings

Ingredients
4 medium unpeeled red potatoes
1 package (8 ounces) sliced fresh mushrooms (3 cups)
3/4 cup chopped fully cooked ham
8 medium green onions, sliced (1/2 cup)
1/8 teaspoon ground red pepper (cayenne)
1/2 cup reduced-fat sour cream
1/2 cup shredded reduced-fat sharp Cheddar cheese (2 ounces)

1 Pierce potatoes with fork. Arrange potatoes about 1 inch apart in circle on microwavable paper towel in microwave oven. Microwave uncovered on High 8 to 10 minutes or until tender. (Or bake potatoes in 375° oven 1 to 1 1/2 hours.) Let potatoes stand until cool enough to handle.

2 While potatoes are cooking, spray 4-quart Dutch oven with cooking spray; heat over medium-high heat. Cook mushrooms in Dutch oven 1 minute, stirring frequently; reduce heat to medium. Cover and cook 3 minutes; remove from heat. Stir in ham, green onions and red pepper. Cover and let stand 4 minutes.

3 Split baked potatoes lengthwise in half; fluff with fork. Spread 1 tablespoon of the sour cream over each potato half. Top with ham mixture and cheese.

1 Serving:

Calories 225
(Calories from Fat 55)
Fat 6g
Saturated Fat 3g
(10% of Calories from
Saturated Fat)
Trans Fat 0g
Cholesterol 25mg
Omega-3 0g
Sodium 560mg

Exchanges:
2 Starch, 1 Vegetable,
1 Very Lean Meat

2 Carbohydrate Choices

Confetti Wild Rice

PREP: 10 min COOK: 55 min
6 servings

Ingredients
1 tablespoon butter
1 1/2 cups sliced fresh mushrooms (4 ounces)
1/2 cup uncooked wild rice
2 medium green onions, thinly sliced (2 tablespoons)
1 1/4 cups water
1/2 teaspoon salt
1/4 teaspoon pepper
1 package (10 ounces) frozen chopped broccoli, thawed and drained
1 tablespoon lemon juice

1   Melt butter in 10-inch nonstick skillet over medium heat.
    Cook mushrooms, wild rice and green onions in butter about
    3 minutes, stirring occasionally, until onions are tender.

2   Stir in water, salt and pepper. Heat to
    boiling, stirring occasionally; reduce heat
    to medium-low. Cover and simmer 40 to
    50 minutes or until rice is tender; drain if
    necessary.

3   Stir in broccoli and lemon juice.
    Cook uncovered about 2 minutes,
    stirring occasionally, until thoroughly
    heated.

1 Serving:

Calories 85
(Calories from Fat 20)
Fat 2g
Saturated Fat 1g
(13% of Calories from
Saturated Fat)
Trans Fat 0g
Cholesterol 5mg
Omega-3 0g
Sodium 220mg

Exchanges:
1 Starch

1 Carbohydrate Choice

Shopping Strategies

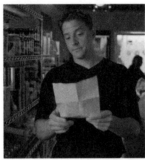

Stick to a grocery list to help prevent impulse buying.

Andersen-Ross/Getty Images

To incorporate healthy choices into your trips to the grocery store, follow these tips:

- Stick to a grocery list to prevent impulse buying.
- Stay in the store's outer aisles, which include the healthy foods (fresh fruits, vegetables, milk, yogurt, fresh meats, fish and poultry, and breads).
- Shop on a full stomach to reduce temptation.
- Buy in-season produce for better taste and price.

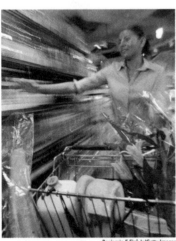

Shop in the outside aisles of grocery stores for healthy foods.

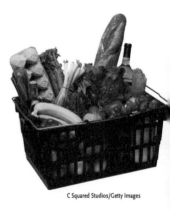

C Squared Studios/Getty Images

Benjamin F Fink Jr/Getty Images

Opportunity is often difficult to recognize; we usually expect it to beckon us with beepers and billboards.
—William Arthur Ward

Notes

MONDAY

Minutes of exercise _____
Weight _____
Blood pressure _____

TUESDAY

Minutes of exercise _____
Weight _____
Blood pressure _____

WEDNESDAY

Minutes of exercise _____
Weight _____
Blood pressure _____

THURSDAY

Minutes of exercise _____
Weight _____
Blood pressure _____

FRIDAY

Minutes of exercise _____
Weight _____
Blood pressure _____

SATURDAY

Minutes of exercise _____
Weight _____
Blood pressure _____

SUNDAY

Minutes of exercise _____
Weight _____
Blood pressure _____

Things to do for next week:

Check next week's supply of:
- ○ vitamins
- ○ blood pressure medication
- ○ diabetes medication
- ○ cholesterol medication
- ○ lancets
- ○ aspirin
- ○ glucose test strips

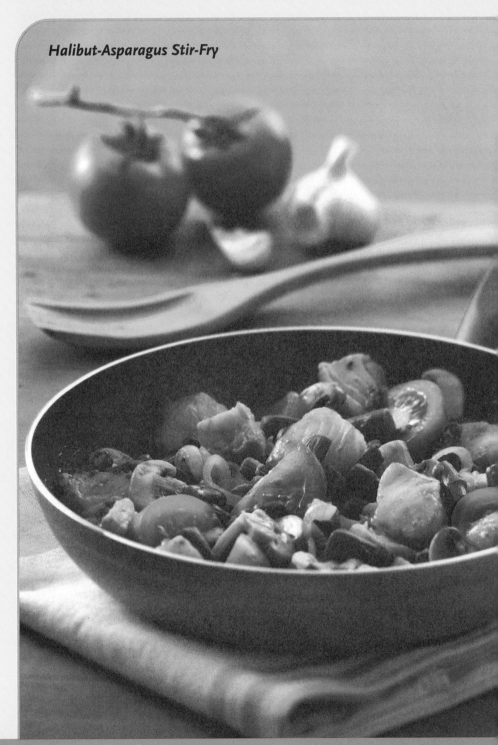

Halibut-Asparagus Stir-Fry

Halibut-Asparagus Stir-Fry

PREP: 10 min COOK: 10 min
4 servings

Ingredients
1 pound halibut, swordfish or tuna fillets, cut into 1-inch pieces
1 medium onion, thinly sliced
1 teaspoon finely chopped gingerroot
3 cloves garlic, finely chopped
1 package (9 ounces) frozen asparagus cuts in a pouch, thawed and drained
1 package (8 ounces) sliced fresh mushrooms (3 cups)
1 medium tomato, cut into thin wedges
2 tablespoons reduced-sodium soy sauce
1 tablespoon lemon juice

1   Spray 10-inch nonstick skillet with cooking spray; heat over
    medium-high heat. Stir-fry fish, onion, gingerroot, garlic and
    asparagus in skillet 2 to 3 minutes or until fish almost flakes
    with fork.

2   Carefully stir in remaining ingredients. Cook 5 to 7 minutes
    or until thoroughly heated and fish flakes easily with fork.
    Serve with additional soy sauce if desired.

1 Serving:

Calories 165
(Calories from Fat 20)
Fat 2g
Saturated Fat 0g
(2% of Calories from
Saturated Fat)
Trans Fat 0g
Cholesterol 60mg
Omega-3 0g
Sodium 370mg

Exchanges:
2 Vegetable,
3 Very Lean Meat

1 Carbohydrate Choice

Talk to Your Pharmacist

Finding it difficult to organize medicines around meals and activities? A pillbox may be helpful. Pillboxes arrange medicines into compartments that let you know whether you have taken your daily dose. If the problem is that you often do not have your medicine with you, try carrying a small pocket- or purse-sized pillbox. Also consider setting alarms on your watch or computer. Some people find it helpful to keep 2 supplies of medicines: 1 at home and 1 at work. Talk to your pharmacist about ideas to simplify taking your medicines.

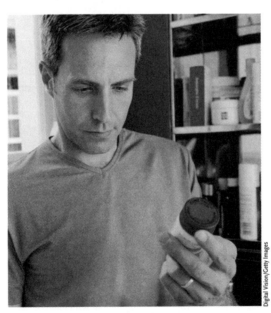

Digital Vision/Getty Images

Check to see how often you need to refill your medications.

Notes

MONDAY

Minutes of exercise _____
Weight _____
Blood pressure _____

TUESDAY

Minutes of exercise _____
Weight _____
Blood pressure _____

WEDNESDAY

Minutes of exercise _____
Weight _____
Blood pressure _____

THURSDAY

Minutes of exercise _____
Weight _____
Blood pressure _____

FRIDAY

Minutes of exercise _____
Weight _____
Blood pressure _____

SATURDAY

Minutes of exercise _____
Weight _____
Blood pressure _____

SUNDAY

Minutes of exercise _____
Weight _____
Blood pressure _____

Things to do for next week:

Check next week's supply of:
- ○ vitamins
- ○ blood pressure medication
- ○ diabetes medication
- ○ cholesterol medication
- ○ lancets
- ○ aspirin
- ○ glucose test strips

Mediterranean Vegetable Salad

PREP: 10 min CHILL: 1 hr
6 servings

Ingredients
1/3 cup tarragon or white wine vinegar
2 tablespoons canola or soybean oil
2 tablespoons chopped fresh or 2 teaspoons dried oregano leaves
1/2 teaspoon sugar
1/2 teaspoon salt
1/2 teaspoon ground mustard
1/2 teaspoon pepper
2 cloves garlic, finely chopped
3 large tomatoes, sliced
2 large yellow bell peppers, sliced into thin rings
6 ounces washed fresh spinach leaves (from 10-ounce bag), stems removed
   (about 1 cup)
1/2 cup crumbled feta cheese (2 ounces)
Kalamata olives, if desired

1   Mix vinegar, oil, oregano, sugar, salt, mustard, pepper and
    garlic in small bowl. Place tomatoes and bell peppers in glass
    or plastic container. Pour vinegar mixture over vegetables.
    Cover and refrigerate at least 1 hour to blend flavors.

2   Line serving platter with spinach.
    Drain vegetables; place on
    spinach. Sprinkle with cheese;
    garnish with olives.

1 Serving:

Calories 120
(Calories from Fat 65)
Fat 7g
Saturated Fat 2g
(14% of Calories from
Saturated Fat)
Trans Fat 0g
Cholesterol 10mg
Omega-3 0g
Sodium 330mg

Exchanges:
2 Vegetable, 1 1/2 Fat

1 Carbohydrate Choice

Fruited Bread Pudding with Eggnog Sauce

PREP: 15 min BAKE: 45 min
8 servings

Ingredients
4 cups 1-inch cubes French bread
1/2 cup diced dried fruit and raisin mixture
2 cups fat-free (skim) milk
1/2 cup fat-free cholesterol-free egg product or 2 eggs
1/3 cup sugar
1/2 teaspoon vanilla
Ground nutmeg, if desired
Eggnog Sauce (below)

1 Serving:

Calories 145
(Calories from Fat 10)
Fat 1g
Saturated Fat 0g
(2% of Calories from
Saturated Fat)
Trans Fat 0g
Cholesterol 0mg
Omega-3 0g
Sodium 190mg

Exchanges:
1/2 Fruit, 1/2 Milk

1 Heat oven to 350°. Spray pie plate, 9 x 1 1/4 inches, with cooking spray. Place bread cubes in pie plate; sprinkle with fruit mixture.

2 Beat milk, egg product, sugar and vanilla in small bowl with wire whisk until smooth. Pour milk mixture over bread. Press bread cubes into milk mixture. Sprinkle with nutmeg.

3 Bake uncovered 40 to 45 minutes or until golden brown and set.

4 Make Eggnog Sauce. Cut bread pudding into wedges, or spoon into serving dishes. Drizzle each serving with scant tablespoon sauce. Sprinkle with additional nutmeg if desired. Store pudding and sauce covered in refrigerator.

Eggnog Sauce
1/3 cup fat-free (skim) milk
1 container (3 to 4 ounces) refrigerated vanilla fat-free pudding
1/2 teaspoon rum extract

Mix all ingredients in small bowl until smooth.

2 Carbohydrate Choices

Cholesterol

Part of a lipid (fats) molecule, cholesterol is a waxlike substance that serves as a building block within the cell membrane. Cholesterol has several functions. It is used to:

- Make hormones like estrogen and testosterone.
- Make bile acids to break down fat in the intestines.

Throughout our lives, lipids can move into the cell wall of the arteries and form fatty streaks, which may turn into plaque. Plaque restricts, or reduces, the flow of blood and increases pressure in the artery.

For a healthier diet, try to limit those foods that are high in cholesterol and saturated fat.

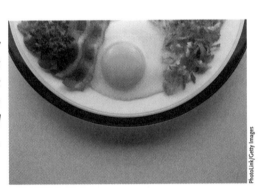

PhotoLink/Getty Images

Notes

MONDAY

Minutes of exercise _____
Weight _____
Blood pressure _____

TUESDAY

Minutes of exercise _____
Weight _____
Blood pressure _____

WEDNESDAY

Minutes of exercise _____
Weight _____
Blood pressure _____

THURSDAY

Minutes of exercise _____
Weight _____
Blood pressure _____

FRIDAY

Minutes of exercise _____
Weight _____
Blood pressure _____

SATURDAY

Minutes of exercise _____
Weight _____
Blood pressure _____

SUNDAY

Minutes of exercise _____
Weight _____
Blood pressure _____

Things to do for next week:

Check next week's supply of:
○ blood pressure medication
○ cholesterol medication
○ aspirin
○ vitamins
○ diabetes medication
○ lancets
○ glucose test strips

White Bean and Spinach Pizza

PREP: 10 min STAND: 10 min BAKE: 10 min
8 servings

Ingredients
1/2 cup sun-dried tomato halves (not oil-packed)
1 can (15 to 16 ounces) great northern or navy beans, rinsed and drained
2 medium cloves garlic, finely chopped
1 package (10 ounces) ready-to-serve thin Italian pizza crust (12 inches
   in diameter)
1/4 teaspoon dried oregano leaves
1 cup firmly packed washed fresh spinach leaves (from 10-ounce bag),
   shredded
1/2 cup shredded reduced-fat Colby-Monterey Jack cheese (2 ounces)

1 Heat oven to 425°. Pour enough boiling water over dried
   tomatoes to cover; let stand 10 minutes. Drain. Cut into thin
   strips; set aside.

2 Place beans and garlic in food processor. Cover and process
   until smooth. Spread beans over pizza crust. Sprinkle with
   oregano, tomatoes, spinach and cheese. Place on ungreased
   cookie sheet.

3 Bake about 10 minutes or until
   cheese is melted.

1 Serving:

Calories 180
(Calories from Fat 25)
Fat 3g
Saturated Fat 1g
(3% of Calories from
Saturated Fat)
Trans Fat 0g
Cholesterol 0mg
Omega-3 0g
Sodium 310mg

Exchanges:
2 Starch, 1/2 Fat

2.5 Carbohydrate Choices

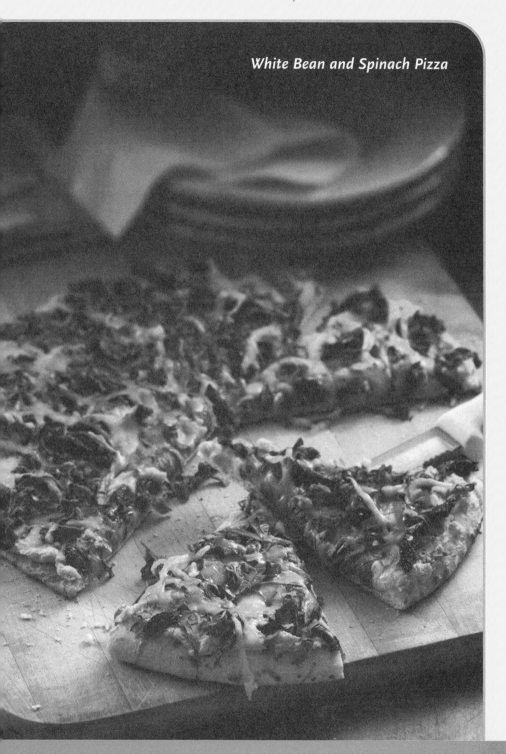

White Bean and Spinach Pizza

Healthy Cooking

There are many healthy and easy ways to cook nutritious foods. Use these healthy cooking methods to prepare your favorite foods at home.

- If you need to use a fat source for food preparation, use olive oil or canola oil.
- Bake, broil, roast, grill, or steam meats, poultry, fish, and vegetables. Trim all skin and visible fat from poultry and meats.
- When baking, replace half of the oil in the recipe with applesauce.
- Replace whole eggs with 2 egg whites. This will help you to save on calories, fat, and cholesterol.
- Rinse cooked ground meat in a colander with warm water. This will remove much of the fat from the meat.
- Use 1% or skim milk and reduced-fat cheeses.

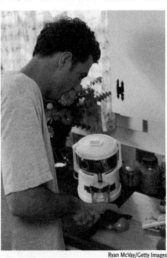

Ryan McVay/Getty Images

Have fruits and vegetables available to provide healthy additions to your meals.

Dollars have never been known to produce character, and character will never be produced by money.
—W.K. Kellogg

Notes

MONDAY

Minutes of exercise _____
Weight _____
Blood pressure _____

TUESDAY

Minutes of exercise _____
Weight _____
Blood pressure _____

WEDNESDAY

Minutes of exercise _____
Weight _____
Blood pressure _____

THURSDAY

Minutes of exercise _____
Weight _____
Blood pressure _____

FRIDAY

Minutes of exercise _____
Weight _____
Blood pressure _____

SATURDAY

Minutes of exercise _____
Weight _____
Blood pressure _____

SUNDAY

Minutes of exercise _____
Weight _____
Blood pressure _____

Things to do for next week:

Check next week's supply of:
- ○ blood pressure medication
- ○ cholesterol medication
- ○ aspirin
- ○ vitamins
- ○ diabetes medication
- ○ lancets
- ○ glucose test strips

Lemon-Date Muffins

PREP: 15 min BAKE: 22 min
12 muffins

Ingredients
1 1/2 cups whole wheat flour
3/4 cup all-purpose flour
3 teaspoons baking powder
1/2 teaspoon salt
1/4 cup packed brown sugar
2 teaspoons grated lemon peel
1 cup fat-free (skim) milk
1/3 cup canola or soybean oil
1 egg
1/2 cup chopped dates

1 Heat oven to 400°. Grease bottoms only of 12 muffin cups with shortening (do not use paper baking cups).

2 Mix flours, baking powder and salt in large bowl; set aside. Beat brown sugar, lemon peel, milk, oil and egg in medium bowl with fork or wire whisk until well mixed. Stir into flour mixture just until flour is moistened. Fold in dates. Divide batter evenly among muffin cups.

3 Bake 18 to 22 minutes or until toothpick inserted in center comes out clean and tops begin to brown. Run knife around edge of cups; remove muffins from pan to wire rack. Serve warm.

1 Muffin:

Calories 195
(Calories from Fat 65)
Fat 7g
Saturated Fat 1g
(3% of Calories from
Saturated Fat)
Trans Fat 0g
Cholesterol 20mg
Omega-3 1g
Sodium 240mg

Exchanges:
1 1/2 Starch, 1/2 Fruit,
1 Fat

2 Carbohydrate Choices

Easy Salmon Spread

PREP: 15 min CHILL: 2 hrs
16 servings (2 tablespoons dip and 4 crackers)

Ingredients
1 package (8 ounces) fat-free cream cheese, softened
1 can (14 3/4 ounces) red or pink salmon, drained and flaked
3 tablespoons finely chopped red onion
2 tablespoons chopped fresh or 1/4 teaspoon dried dill weed
1 tablespoon Dijon mustard
2 tablespoons capers
64 reduced-fat whole-grain crackers

1 Line 2-cup bowl or mold with plastic wrap. Beat cream cheese in medium bowl with electric mixer on medium speed until smooth. Stir in salmon, 2 tablespoons of the red onion, 1 tablespoon of the dill weed and the mustard.

2 Spoon into bowl lined with plastic wrap, pressing firmly. Cover and refrigerate at least 2 hours but no longer than 24 hours.

3 Turn bowl upside down onto serving plate; remove bowl and plastic wrap. Garnish with remaining 1 tablespoon red onion, 1 tablespoon dill weed and the capers. Serve with crackers.

1 Serving:

Calories 115
(Calories from Fat 25)
Fat 3g
Saturated Fat 1g
(8% of Calories from
Saturated Fat)
Trans Fat 0g
Cholesterol 15mg
Omega-3 0g
Sodium 380mg

Exchanges:
1 Starch, 1 Very
Lean Meat

1 Carbohydrate Choice

Omega-3 Fatty Acids

Omega-3 fatty acids are essential fatty acids. The body cannot manufacture them; therefore, they need to be obtained through diet. Omega-3 fatty acids have many benefits. They have been shown to:

- Decrease blood clots
- Lower blood pressure
- Decrease cholesterol and triglyceride levels

The American Heart Association recommends 2 to 3 servings of fish — specifically salmon, albacore tuna, herring, bluefish, lake trout, mackerel, and sardines — per week to obtain sufficient amounts of omega-3 fats. Nuts, seeds, and flaxseed oil are also significant sources of omega-3 fatty acids.

Due to an increased risk of excessive mercury exposure in some fish, children and pregnant or nursing women should speak to a doctor before consuming fish.

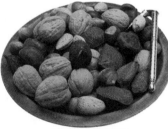

C Squared Studios/Getty Images

Adding nuts and seeds to salads is a simple way of adding omega-3 fatty acids to your diet.

Not everything that is faced can be changed, but nothing can be changed until it is faced.
—James Baldwin

Notes

MONDAY

Minutes of exercise _____
Weight _____
Blood pressure _____

TUESDAY

Minutes of exercise _____
Weight _____
Blood pressure _____

WEDNESDAY

Minutes of exercise _____
Weight _____
Blood pressure _____

THURSDAY

Minutes of exercise _____
Weight _____
Blood pressure _____

FRIDAY

Minutes of exercise _____
Weight _____
Blood pressure _____

SATURDAY

Minutes of exercise _____
Weight _____
Blood pressure _____

SUNDAY

Minutes of exercise _____
Weight _____
Blood pressure _____

Things to do for next week:

Check next week's supply of:
- ○ blood pressure medication
- ○ cholesterol medication
- ○ aspirin
- ○ vitamins
- ○ diabetes medication
- ○ lancets
- ○ glucose test strips

Peach and Blueberry Crisp with Crunchy Topping

PREP: 20 min BAKE: 30 min
6 servings

Ingredients
4 medium peaches, peeled and sliced (2 3/4 cups)
1 cup fresh or frozen (thawed and drained) blueberries
2 tablespoons packed brown sugar
2 tablespoons orange juice
1 teaspoon ground cinnamon
1/4 teaspoon ground nutmeg
1 cup Honey Nut Clusters® cereal, slightly crushed
1/3 cup chopped pecans
3/4 cup frozen (thawed) fat-free whipped topping

1 Heat oven to 375°. Spray bottom and sides of square baking dish, 8 x 8 x 2 inches, or rectangular baking dish, 11 x 7 x 1 1/2 inches, with cooking spray.

2 Place peaches and blueberries in baking dish. Mix brown sugar, orange juice, cinnamon and nutmeg in small bowl; drizzle over fruit.

3 Bake 15 minutes. Sprinkle with crushed cereal and pecans. Bake 10 to 15 minutes longer or until peaches are tender when pierced with a fork. Serve warm or cold with whipped topping.

1 Serving:

Calories 170
(Calories from Fat 55)
Fat 6g
Saturated Fat 1g
(4% of Calories from Saturated Fat)
Trans Fat 0g
Cholesterol 0mg
Omega-3 0g
Sodium 50mg

Exchanges:
1 Starch, 1 Fruit, 1 Fat

2 Carbohydrate Choices

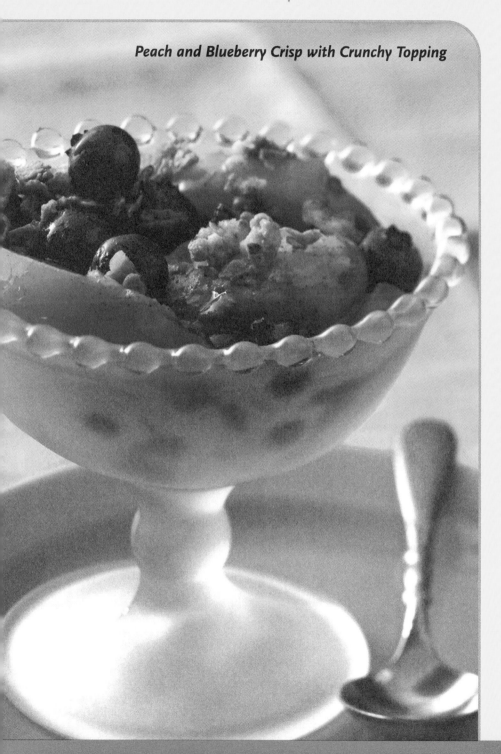

Peach and Blueberry Crisp with Crunchy Topping

Over-the-Counter Items

Be careful when taking over-the-counter medicines and vitamins. Some of these can cause drug interactions. Existing medical conditions, exercise, tobacco, alcohol, and other medicines can all cause interactions with over-the-counter medications.

To avoid drug interactions, always:

- Check with your doctor or pharmacist before taking a new medicine.
- Tell your doctor and pharmacist about all prescription and over-the-counter medicines, nutritional supplements, and vitamins you are taking.

Talk to your pharmacist before you purchase over-the-counter medicines. Be sure they will not interact with your current medications.

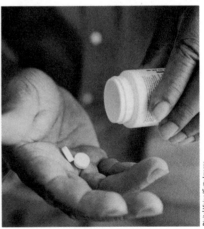

Digital Vision/Getty Images

Mistakes are the usual bridge between experience and wisdom.
—Phyllis Theroux

Notes

MONDAY

Minutes of exercise _____
Weight _____
Blood pressure _____

TUESDAY

Minutes of exercise _____
Weight _____
Blood pressure _____

WEDNESDAY

Minutes of exercise _____
Weight _____
Blood pressure _____

THURSDAY

Minutes of exercise _____
Weight _____
Blood pressure _____

FRIDAY

Minutes of exercise _____
Weight _____
Blood pressure _____

SATURDAY

Minutes of exercise _____
Weight _____
Blood pressure _____

SUNDAY

Minutes of exercise _____
Weight _____
Blood pressure _____

Things to do for next week:

Check next week's supply of:
- ○ blood pressure medication
- ○ cholesterol medication
- ○ aspirin
- ○ vitamins
- ○ diabetes medication
- ○ lancets
- ○ glucose test strips

Baked Fish with Italian Rice

PREP: 25 min BAKE: 25 min
6 servings

Ingredients
2 tablespoons water
1 medium onion, chopped (1/2 cup)
3 cups cooked brown or white rice
1 can (14 1/2 ounces) no-salt-added Italian-style stewed tomatoes, undrained
1 teaspoon Italian seasoning, crumbled
6 mackerel, snapper, tilapia, sturgeon or any fish fillets, 1/4 inch thick (about 1 pound)
1 1/2 teaspoons canola or soybean oil
1/2 teaspoon paprika

1 Heat oven to 400°. Heat water to boiling in 2 1/2-quart saucepan over medium-high heat. Cook onion in water, stirring occasionally, until crisp-tender. Stir in rice, tomatoes and Italian seasoning; cook until thoroughly heated.

2 Spoon rice mixture into ungreased rectangular baking dish, 13 x 9 x 2 inches. Place fish fillets on rice mixture. Brush fish with oil. Sprinkle with paprika.

3 Cover and bake 20 to 25 minutes or until fish flakes easily with fork.

1 Serving:

Calories 245
(Calories from Fat 65)
Fat 7g
Saturated Fat 1g
(4% of Calories from Saturated Fat)
Trans Fat 0g
Cholesterol 40mg
Omega-3 2g
Sodium 45mg

Exchanges:
1 1/2 Starch, 1 Vegetable, 2 Lean Meat

2 Carbohydrate Choices

Glazed Chicken over Couscous Pilaf

PREP: 10 min COOK: 2 min STAND: 5 min BROIL: 10 min
2 servings

Ingredients
Couscous Pilaf (below)
2 tablespoons orange juice
1 tablespoon apricot preserves or honey
1/2 teaspoon spicy brown mustard
2 boneless skinless chicken breast halves

1 Serving:

Calories 360
(Calories from Fat 35)
Fat 4g
Saturated Fat 1g
(3% of Calories from
Saturated Fat)
Trans Fat 0g
Cholesterol 75mg
Omega-3 0g
Sodium 260mg

Exchanges:
2 Starch, 1 Fruit,
4 Very Lean Meat

1 Make Couscous Pilaf. Set oven control to broil. Mix orange juice, preserves and mustard in small bowl. Pour half of mixture (about 2 tablespoons) into another small dish; reserve for topping.

2 Place chicken on rack in broiler pan; brush with about half of remaining orange juice glaze.

3 Broil with tops about 4 inches from heat 8 to 10 minutes, turning and brushing with glaze after 5 minutes, until juice of chicken is no longer pink when centers of thickest pieces are cut. Discard any remaining glaze.

4 Stir pilaf lightly with fork; divide evenly onto plates. Top with chicken; drizzle with reserved orange juice mixture.

Couscous Pilaf

1/2 cup frozen sweet peas	1/8 teaspoon ground ginger
3/4 cup water	1/2 cup uncooked couscous

Place peas, water and ginger in 1-quart saucepan. Heat to boiling over high heat; reduce heat to medium-low. Cover and simmer 2 minutes. Remove from heat; stir in couscous. Cover; let stand 5 minutes.

3 Carbohydrate Choices

What to Eat

Improve your overall diet by eating a variety of healthy foods. The American Heart Association recommends increasing whole grains, such as whole wheat breads and whole grain cereals, and eating at least 5 servings of fruits and vegetables every day.

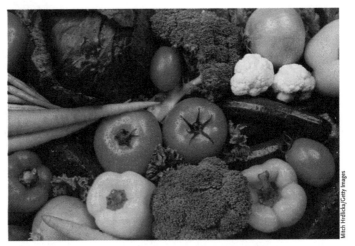

Try eating a balanced diet that includes 5 servings of fruit and/or vegetables per day.

Notes

MONDAY

Minutes of exercise _____
Weight _____
Blood pressure _____

TUESDAY

Minutes of exercise _____
Weight _____
Blood pressure _____

WEDNESDAY

Minutes of exercise _____
Weight _____
Blood pressure _____

THURSDAY

Minutes of exercise _____
Weight _____
Blood pressure _____

FRIDAY

Minutes of exercise _____
Weight _____
Blood pressure _____

SATURDAY

Minutes of exercise _____
Weight _____
Blood pressure _____

SUNDAY

Minutes of exercise _____
Weight _____
Blood pressure _____

Things to do for next week:

Check next week's supply of:
- ○ blood pressure medication
- ○ cholesterol medication
- ○ aspirin
- ○ vitamins
- ○ diabetes medication
- ○ lancets
- ○ glucose test strips

Polenta with Italian Vegetables

PREP: 15 min COOK: 20 min
6 servings

Ingredients
1 cup whole-grain yellow cornmeal
3/4 cup cold water
2 1/2 cups boiling water
1/2 teaspoon salt
2/3 cup shredded Swiss cheese
2 teaspoons canola or soybean oil
4 medium zucchini or yellow summer squash, sliced (about 4 cups)
1 medium red bell pepper, chopped (1 cup)
1 small onion, chopped (1/4 cup)
1 clove garlic, finely chopped
1/4 cup chopped fresh or 1 tablespoon dried basil leaves
1 can (about 14 ounces) artichoke hearts, drained

1 Beat cornmeal and cold water in 2-quart saucepan with
   wire whisk. Stir in boiling water and salt. Cook over
   medium-high heat, stirring constantly, until mixture thickens
   and boils; reduce heat. Cover and simmer 10 minutes,
   stirring occasionally. Stir in cheese until smooth; keep
   polenta warm.

2 Heat oil in 10-inch nonstick skillet over medium-high heat.
   Cook zucchini, bell pepper, onion and garlic in oil about
   5 minutes, stirring occasionally, until vegetables are
   crisp-tender. Stir in basil and artichoke hearts. Serve
   vegetable mixture over polenta.

2.5 Carbohydrate Choices

Polenta with Italian Vegetables

1 Serving:

Calories 185
(Calories from Fat 55)
Fat 6g
Saturated Fat 2g
(11% of Calories from
Saturated Fat)
Trans Fat 0g
Cholesterol 10mg
Omega-3 0g
Sodium 430mg

Exchanges:
1 Starch, 3 Vegetable,
1 Fat

Aerobic Exercise

It is important to exercise at a level that benefits your cardiovascular system. Things to consider include:

- Type of exercise
- Amount and regularity of exercise
- Intensity of exercise

Consult your doctor about the right type and duration of exercise prior to beginning an exercise routine.

The best type of exercise is aerobic — like walking, jogging, cycling, swimming, cross-country skiing, and rowing — which requires a lot of oxygen.

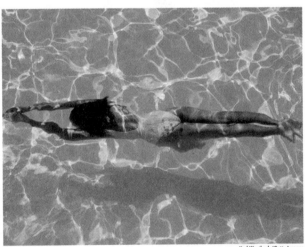

Karl Weatherly/Getty Images

Find at least 1 exercise you can maintain as part of a daily routine.

Notes

MONDAY

Minutes of exercise _____
Weight _____
Blood pressure _____

TUESDAY

Minutes of exercise _____
Weight _____
Blood pressure _____

WEDNESDAY

Minutes of exercise _____
Weight _____
Blood pressure _____

THURSDAY

Minutes of exercise _____
Weight _____
Blood pressure _____

FRIDAY

Minutes of exercise _____
Weight _____
Blood pressure _____

SATURDAY

Minutes of exercise _____
Weight _____
Blood pressure _____

SUNDAY

Minutes of exercise _____
Weight _____
Blood pressure _____

Things to do for next week:

Check next week's supply of:
○ vitamins
○ blood pressure medication
○ diabetes medication
○ cholesterol medication
○ lancets
○ aspirin
○ glucose test strips

Garbanzo Bean Sandwiches

PREP: 15 min
8 servings

Ingredients
1 can (15 to 16 ounces) garbanzo beans, rinsed and drained
1/2 cup water
2 tablespoons chopped fresh parsley
2 tablespoons chopped walnuts
1 tablespoon finely chopped onion
1 clove garlic, finely chopped
1/2 medium cucumber, sliced
4 whole-wheat pita breads (6 inches in diameter)
Lettuce leaves
1 medium tomato, seeded and chopped (3/4 cup)
1/2 cup cucumber ranch dressing

1   Place beans, water, parsley, walnuts, onion and garlic in food
    processor or blender. Cover and process until smooth.

2   Cut cucumber slices into fourths. Cut each pita bread in
    half to form 2 pockets; line with lettuce leaves. Spoon
    2 tablespoons bean mixture into each pita half. Add tomato,
    cucumber and dressing.

1 Serving:

Calories 225
(Calories from Fat 90)
Fat 10g
Saturated Fat 1g
(4% of Calories from
Saturated Fat)
Trans Fat 0g
Cholesterol 5mg
Omega-3 1g
Sodium 370mg

Exchanges:
2 Starch, 1/2 Lean Meat,
1 Fat

2 Carbohydrate Choices

Mexican Rice and Bean Bake

PREP: 10 min COOK: 10 min BAKE: 35 min STAND: 5 min
6 servings

Ingredients
1 1/4 cups water
1 cup uncooked instant brown rice
1 1/2 cups picante sauce
1 cup shredded reduced-fat Cheddar cheese (4 ounces)
1/4 cup fat-free cholesterol-free egg product or 1 egg
1 can (15 to 16 ounces) pinto beans, drained
1/4 teaspoon chili powder

1   Heat water to boiling in 1-quart saucepan. Stir in rice; reduce heat to low. Cover and simmer 10 minutes. Meanwhile, heat oven to 350°. Spray square baking dish, 8 x 8 x 2 inches, with cooking spray.

2   Mix rice, 1/2 cup of the picante sauce, 1/2 cup of the cheese and the egg product in medium bowl; press in bottom of baking dish.

3   Mix beans and remaining 1 cup picante sauce in small bowl; spoon over rice mixture. Sprinkle with remaining 1/2 cup cheese and the chili powder.

4   Bake uncovered 30 to 35 minutes or until cheese is melted and bubbly. Let stand 5 minutes before serving.

1 Serving:

Calories 195
(Calories from Fat 20)
Fat 2g
Saturated Fat 1g
(4% of Calories from Saturated Fat)
Trans Fat 0g
Cholesterol 5mg
Omega-3 0g
Sodium 620mg

Exchanges:
2 Starch, 1 Vegetable

2.5 Carbohydrate Choices

Exercise Tips

When you are just starting out, try to exercise very comfortably. Here are 3 quick tips.

1) Try to exercise so that you are breathing noticeably but are not out of breath. Remember this simple rule: you should be able to carry on a conversation while you are exercising.

2) Sweating is a good thing. This means that your muscles are working hard enough to generate heat and improve fitness. Sweat is the body's protective mechanism to cool itself.

3) If you are not fatigued and are completely recovered from exercising on the previous day, then you should exercise daily.

Be sure you remain properly hydrated during your exercise.

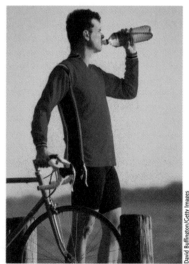

David Buffington/Getty Images

Notes

MONDAY

Minutes of exercise _____
Weight _____
Blood pressure _____

TUESDAY

Minutes of exercise _____
Weight _____
Blood pressure _____

WEDNESDAY

Minutes of exercise _____
Weight _____
Blood pressure _____

THURSDAY

Minutes of exercise _____
Weight _____
Blood pressure _____

FRIDAY

Minutes of exercise _____
Weight _____
Blood pressure _____

SATURDAY

Minutes of exercise _____
Weight _____
Blood pressure _____

SUNDAY

Minutes of exercise _____
Weight _____
Blood pressure _____

Things to do for next week:

Check next week's supply of:
○ blood pressure medication
○ cholesterol medication
○ aspirin
○ vitamins
○ diabetes medication
○ lancets
○ glucose test strips

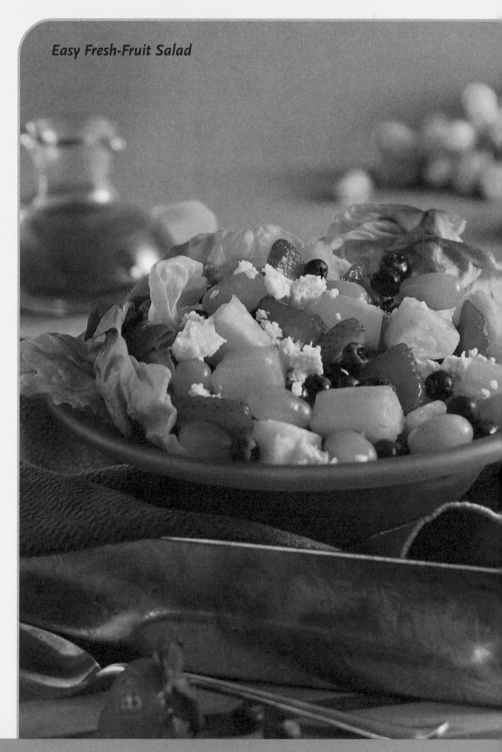

Easy Fresh-Fruit Salad

Easy Fresh-Fruit Salad

PREP: 20 min
6 servings

Ingredients
1 medium pineapple (2 pounds), peeled and cut into 1-inch chunks (3 cups)
1 pint (2 cups) fresh strawberries, sliced
1 pint (2 cups) fresh blueberries
2 cups seedless green grapes
1 bunch leaf lettuce
1/2 cup raspberry vinaigrette dressing
3/4 to 1 cup crumbled feta cheese (3 to 4 ounces)

1 Mix pineapple, strawberries, blueberries and grapes in large bowl.

2 Line individual serving plates with lettuce; spoon salad onto lettuce. Drizzle with dressing; sprinkle with cheese.

1 Serving:

Calories 170
(Calories from Fat 35)
Fat 4g
Saturated Fat 2g
(12% of Calories from
Saturated Fat)
Trans Fat 0g
Cholesterol 15mg
Omega-3 0g
Sodium 400mg

Exchanges:
2 Fruit, 1/2 High-Fat Meat

2 Carbohydrate Choices

Blood Pressure

Several factors may contribute to high blood pressure (hypertension) and cardiovascular disease. These include:

- Excess dietary salt
- Excess alcohol intake
- Stress
- Age
- Genetics and family history
- Obesity
- Physical inactivity
- High saturated fat diet
- Smoking

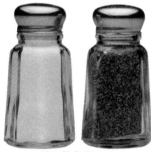

C Squared Studios/Getty Images

The American Heart Association recommends people consume 2,400 mg or less of sodium per day. Ask a registered dietitian how to limit salt intake.

Notes

MONDAY

Minutes of exercise _____
Weight _____
Blood pressure _____

TUESDAY

Minutes of exercise _____
Weight _____
Blood pressure _____

WEDNESDAY

Minutes of exercise _____
Weight _____
Blood pressure _____

THURSDAY

Minutes of exercise _____
Weight _____
Blood pressure _____

FRIDAY

Minutes of exercise _____
Weight _____
Blood pressure _____

SATURDAY

Minutes of exercise _____
Weight _____
Blood pressure _____

SUNDAY

Minutes of exercise _____
Weight _____
Blood pressure _____

Things to do for next week:

Check next week's supply of:
- ○ blood pressure medication
- ○ cholesterol medication
- ○ aspirin
- ○ vitamins
- ○ diabetes medication
- ○ lancets
- ○ glucose test strips

Corn and Black Bean Salad

PREP: 5 min   CHILL: 2 hr
6 servings

Ingredients
1 can (15 ounces) black beans, rinsed and drained
1 can (about 8 ounces) whole kernel corn, drained
1 can (4 1/2 ounces) chopped green chiles, drained
1/2 cup medium chunky-style salsa
1/4 cup chopped onion
2 tablespoons chopped fresh cilantro

Mix all ingredients in medium bowl. Cover and refrigerate until chilled, at least 2 hours but no longer than 24 hours.

1 Serving:

Calories 135
(Calories from Fat 10)
Fat 1g
Saturated Fat 0g
(1% of Calories from Saturated Fat)
Trans Fat 0g
Cholesterol 0mg
Omega-3 0g
Sodium 800mg

Exchanges:
2 Starch

2 Carbohydrate Choices

Fruit with Caramel Sauce

PREP: 10 min
6 servings

Ingredients
1 medium nectarine or peach, pitted and cut into wedges
1 kiwifruit, peeled and sliced
1 cup fresh strawberries, halved
1 cup fresh blueberries
2/3 cup caramel ice cream topping
1/4 teaspoon rum extract

1   Arrange fruit on individual dessert plates or in dessert dishes.

2   Mix ice cream topping and rum extract in 1-quart saucepan;
    heat over medium heat, stirring occasionally, until warm.
    Drizzle 1 heaping tablespoon topping mixture over each
    serving of fruit.

1 Serving:

Calories 140
(Calories from Fat 0)
Fat 0g
Saturated Fat 0g
(2% of Calories from
Saturated Fat)
Trans Fat 0g
Cholesterol 0mg
Omega-3 0g
Sodium 130mg

Exchanges:
2 1/2 Fruit

2 Carbohydrate Choices

Safe Medication Use

Follow these tips for safe use of your medication(s):

- Read package directions and warnings.
- Tell all care providers about all medicines.
- Use a single pharmacy for all prescriptions.
- Know both generic and brand names of your medicines.
- Understand how medicines work.
- Know your correct dose and proper use.
- Be aware of possible side effects.
- Keep a list of all current prescription and nonprescription medicines.

Be sure to read the labels on your medicines. Be aware of the possible side effects.

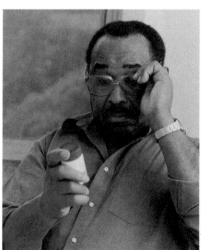

Digital Vision/Getty Images

Notes

MONDAY

Minutes of exercise _____
Weight _____
Blood pressure _____

TUESDAY

Minutes of exercise _____
Weight _____
Blood pressure _____

WEDNESDAY

Minutes of exercise _____
Weight _____
Blood pressure _____

THURSDAY

Minutes of exercise _____
Weight _____
Blood pressure _____

FRIDAY

Minutes of exercise _____
Weight _____
Blood pressure _____

SATURDAY

Minutes of exercise _____
Weight _____
Blood pressure _____

SUNDAY

Minutes of exercise _____
Weight _____
Blood pressure _____

Things to do for next week:

Check next week's supply of:
- ○ blood pressure medication
- ○ cholesterol medication
- ○ aspirin
- ○ vitamins
- ○ diabetes medication
- ○ lancets
- ○ glucose test strips

Caramelized Onion and Sweet Potato Skillet

PREP: 10 min COOK: 20 min
4 servings

Ingredients
1 teaspoon canola or soybean oil
3 medium sweet potatoes (about 1 pound), peeled and sliced (about
  3 1/2 cups)
1/4 large sweet onion (Bermuda, Maui, Spanish or Walla Walla), sliced
2 tablespoons packed brown sugar
1/2 teaspoon jerk seasoning (dry)
1 tablespoon chopped fresh parsley

1 Heat oil in 10-inch skillet over medium heat. Cook sweet
   potatoes and onion in oil about 5 minutes, stirring
   occasionally, until light brown; reduce heat to low. Cover
   and cook 10 to 12 minutes, stirring occasionally, until
   potatoes are tender.

2 Stir in brown sugar and jerk seasoning. Cook uncovered
   about 3 minutes, stirring occasionally, until glazed.
   Sprinkle with parsley.

1 Serving:

Calories 115
(Calories from Fat 10)
Fat 1g
Saturated Fat 0g
(1% of Calories from
Saturated Fat)
Trans Fat 0g
Cholesterol 0mg
Omega-3 0g
Sodium 10mg

Exchanges:
1/2 Starch, 1 Fruit,
1 Vegetable

2.5 Carbohydrate Choices

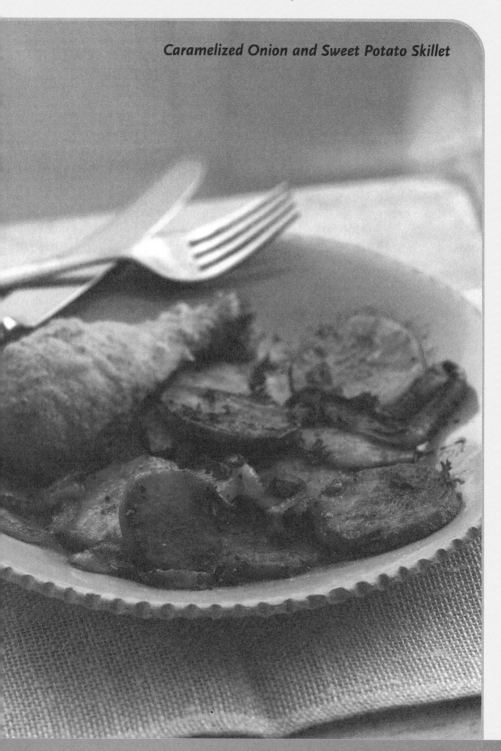

Caramelized Onion and Sweet Potato Skillet

Obesity

Obesity increases the risk of both heart disease and diabetes. Obesity may:

- Raise triglycerides
- Lower HDL-cholesterol
- Raise LDL-cholesterol
- Raise blood pressure

Obesity occurs when the calories we consume exceed the calories we burn through regular activities and exercise.

Maintaining an active lifestyle has many potential benefits and may reduce the risk of complications associated with heart disease and diabetes.

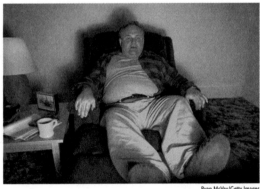

Ryan McVay/Getty Images

Notes

MONDAY

Minutes of exercise _____
Weight _____
Blood pressure _____

TUESDAY

Minutes of exercise _____
Weight _____
Blood pressure _____

WEDNESDAY

Minutes of exercise _____
Weight _____
Blood pressure _____

THURSDAY

Minutes of exercise _____
Weight _____
Blood pressure _____

FRIDAY

Minutes of exercise _____
Weight _____
Blood pressure _____

SATURDAY

Minutes of exercise _____
Weight _____
Blood pressure _____

SUNDAY

Minutes of exercise _____
Weight _____
Blood pressure _____

Things to do for next week:

Check next week's supply of:
- ○ blood pressure medication
- ○ cholesterol medication
- ○ aspirin
- ○ vitamins
- ○ diabetes medication
- ○ lancets
- ○ glucose test strips

Canadian Bacon and Potato Frittata

PREP: 10 min COOK: 23 min
4 servings

Ingredients
1 1/2 cups fat-free cholesterol-free egg product or 6 eggs
2 tablespoons chopped fresh chives or 1 tablespoon freeze-dried chopped
  chives
2 tablespoons fat-free (skim) milk
1/4 teaspoon salt
1/8 teaspoon dried thyme leaves
1/8 teaspoon pepper
1/4 cup chopped red or green bell pepper
2 cups refrigerated southern-style hash-brown potatoes
1/2 cup coarsely chopped Canadian bacon or cooked ham
2 tablespoons shredded Cheddar cheese

1 Beat egg product, chives, milk, salt, thyme and pepper in medium bowl; set aside.

2 Spray 10-inch nonstick skillet with cooking spray. Add bell pepper; cook and stir over medium heat 1 minute. Add potatoes; cover and cook 8 to 10 minutes, stirring frequently until potatoes begin to brown. Stir in Canadian bacon; cook and stir 1 to 2 minutes or until thoroughly heated.

3 Add egg mixture to skillet; cover and cook over medium-low heat until set, 6 to 9 minutes, lifting edges occasionally to allow uncooked egg mixture to flow to bottom of skillet.

4 Sprinkle with cheese. Cover; cook until cheese is melted, about 1 minute longer. Cut into wedges.

1 Serving:

Calories 215
(Calories from Fat 25)
Fat 3g
(Saturated 1g)
Trans Fat 0g
Cholesterol 15mg
Omega-3 0g
Sodium 610mg

Exchanges:
2 Starch, 2 Very Lean
Meat

2 Carbohydrate Choices

Hummus-Olive Spread

PREP: 10 min COOK: 23 min
10 servings (2 tablespoons spread and 4 pita wedges each)

Ingredients
1 container (7 ounces) plain hummus, or Hummus (below)
1/2 cup pitted Kalamata and/or Spanish olives, chopped or 1 can
    (4 1/4 ounces) chopped ripe olives, drained
1 tablespoon Greek vinaigrette or zesty fat-free Italian dressing
7 pita breads (6 inches in diameter), each cut into 6 wedges

1 Spread hummus on 8- to 10-inch serving
plate.

2 Mix olives and vinaigrette in small bowl.
Spoon over hummus. Serve with pita bread
wedges.

Hummus
1/2 can (15 to 16 ounces) garbanzo beans, drained and
    2 tablespoons liquid reserved
2 tablespoons lemon juice
1/4 cup sesame seed
1 small clove garlic, crushed
1/2 teaspoon salt

Place all ingredients including reserved bean
liquid in blender or food processor. Cover
and blend on high speed, stopping blender
occasionally to scrape sides if necessary, until
uniform consistency.

1 Serving:

Calories 154
(Calories from Fat 28)
Fat 4g
Saturated Fat 0g
(1% of Calories from
Saturated Fat)
Trans Fat 0g
Cholesterol 0mg
Omega-3 0g
Sodium 340mg

Exchanges:
1 1/2 Starch, 1/2 Fat

1.5 Carbohydrate Choices

Metabolic Syndrome

Metabolic syndrome affects 1 of every 4 Americans (2 of every 5 people over age 60). Individuals who have at least 3 of the following criteria are considered to have this condition:

1) Abdominal obesity (large waist girth)
2) Elevated triglyceride levels
3) Low HDL-cholesterol
4) High blood pressure
5) Fasting blood glucose levels greater than 100 mg/dL.

Those with metabolic syndrome are at increased risk for heart attack, stroke or even death.

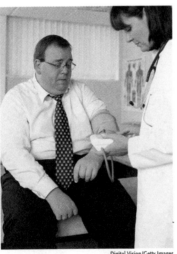

Digital Vision/Getty Images

People who have metabolic syndrome may also be at increased risk of heart disease.

Notes

MONDAY

Minutes of exercise _____
Weight _____
Blood pressure _____

TUESDAY

Minutes of exercise _____
Weight _____
Blood pressure _____

WEDNESDAY

Minutes of exercise _____
Weight _____
Blood pressure _____

THURSDAY

Minutes of exercise _____
Weight _____
Blood pressure _____

FRIDAY

Minutes of exercise _____
Weight _____
Blood pressure _____

SATURDAY

Minutes of exercise _____
Weight _____
Blood pressure _____

SUNDAY

Minutes of exercise _____
Weight _____
Blood pressure _____

Things to do for next week:

Check next week's supply of:
- ○ blood pressure medication
- ○ cholesterol medication
- ○ aspirin
- ○ vitamins
- ○ diabetes medication
- ○ lancets
- ○ glucose test strips

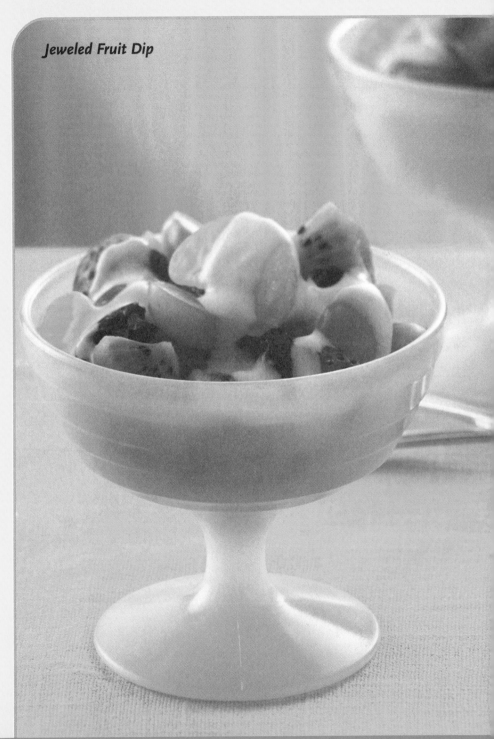

Jeweled Fruit Dip

Jeweled Fruit Dip

PREP: 15 min
8 servings

Ingredients
1 cup vanilla low-fat yogurt
1 tablespoon mayonnaise or salad dressing
1/4 teaspoon grated orange or lemon peel
2 tablespoons orange or lemon juice
1 pint strawberries (2 cups), sliced
1 1/2 cups seedless green grapes, cut in half
1 medium kiwifruit, peeled and chopped
1 can (11 ounces) mandarin orange segments, drained
3 tablespoons dried cranberries

1 Mix yogurt, mayonnaise, orange peel and orange juice in small bowl; set aside.

2 Mix remaining ingredients in large bowl. Serve with yogurt mixture.

1 Serving:

Calories 90
(Calories from Fat 20)
Fat 2g
Saturated Fat 0g
(4% of Calories from
Saturated Fat)
Trans Fat 0g
Cholesterol 0mg
Omega-3 0g
Sodium 30mg

Exchanges:
1 1/2 Fruit, 1/2 Fat

3 Carbohydrate Choices

Reducing Heart Risks

After a heart attack, bypass surgery, or angioplasty, you can take steps to reduce the risk of future problems. Stay in close contact with your doctor, who might advise you to:

- Stop smoking.
- Take a beta blocker drug and/or an enteric-coated aspirin.
- Keep LDL-cholesterol below 70 mg/dL with drugs called "statins."
- Follow a "heart-healthy diet."
- Start exercising (mainly walking).

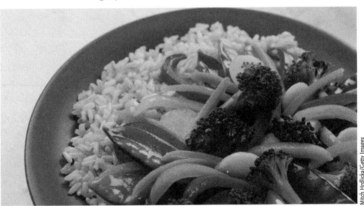

Talk to a dietitian for recommendations on how to prepare "heart healthy" meals.

Notes

MONDAY

Minutes of exercise _____
Weight _____
Blood pressure _____

TUESDAY

Minutes of exercise _____
Weight _____
Blood pressure _____

WEDNESDAY

Minutes of exercise _____
Weight _____
Blood pressure _____

THURSDAY

Minutes of exercise _____
Weight _____
Blood pressure _____

FRIDAY

Minutes of exercise _____
Weight _____
Blood pressure _____

SATURDAY

Minutes of exercise _____
Weight _____
Blood pressure _____

SUNDAY

Minutes of exercise _____
Weight _____
Blood pressure _____

Things to do for next week:

Check next week's supply of:
- ○ blood pressure medication
- ○ cholesterol medication
- ○ aspirin
- ○ vitamins
- ○ diabetes medication
- ○ lancets
- ○ glucose test strips

Tuna Steaks with Fruit Salsa

PREP: 15 min   BROIL: 10 min
2 servings

Ingredients
Fruit Salsa (below)
1 tablespoon packed brown sugar
1 tablespoon fresh lime juice
2 swordfish, tuna or halibut steaks, 3/4 inch thick (4 ounces each)

1 Serving:

Calories 154
(Calories from Fat 28)
Fat 4g
Saturated Fat 0g
(1% of Calories from
Saturated Fat)
Trans Fat 0g
Cholesterol 0mg
Omega-3 0g
Sodium 340mg

Exchanges:
1 1/2 Fruit,
3 Very Lean Meat, 1/2 Fat

1 Make Fruit Salsa. Set oven control to broil. Spray broiler pan rack with cooking spray.

2 Mix brown sugar and lime juice in small bowl. Arrange tuna steaks on rack in broiler pan. Brush with brown sugar mixture.

3 Broil with tops 4 to 6 inches from heat 4 to 5 minutes on each side or until fish flakes easily with fork, brushing occasionally with brown sugar mixture. Serve fish with salsa.

Fruit Salsa
1 tablespoon chopped red onion
2 teaspoons chopped fresh cilantro
1 can (11 ounces) pineapple and mandarin orange
    segments, drained, coarsely chopped
1/2 to 1 jalapeño chili, seeded, chopped (2 to
    3 teaspoons)
2 teaspoons lime juice
1/8 teaspoon salt

Mix ingredients in medium microwavable bowl. Microwave on High 1 1/2 to 2 minutes, stirring once, until thoroughly heated. Cover to keep warm.

1.5 Carbohydrate Choices

Honey-Mustard Chicken and Carrots

PREP: 5 min COOK: 23 min
4 servings

Ingredients
2 teaspoons canola or soybean oil
4 boneless skinless chicken breast halves
1/2 cup apple juice
2 cups frozen baby-cut carrots
2 tablespoons sweet honey mustard
3 tablespoons coarsely chopped honey-roasted peanuts

1 Heat oil in 10-inch nonstick skillet over medium-high heat. Cook chicken in hot oil 5 to 8 minutes or until chicken is browned on both sides.

2 Add apple juice; reduce heat to medium. Cover and cook 5 minutes. Add carrots; cover and cook 5 to 10 minutes or until juice of chicken is no longer pink when centers of thickest pieces are cut and carrots are crisp-tender.

3 Remove chicken and carrots from skillet with slotted spoon; cover to keep warm. Stir mustard into liquid in skillet. Spoon mustard sauce over chicken and carrots. Sprinkle with peanuts.

1 Serving:

Calories 280
(Calories from Fat 90)
Fat 10g
Saturated Fat 2g
(6% of Calories from
Saturated Fat)
Trans Fat 0g
Cholesterol 70mg
Omega-3 0g
Sodium 160mg

Exchanges:
1 Starch, 1 Vegetable,
3 Lean Meat

1 Carbohydrate Choice

Saturated Fat

You can easily decrease the amount of saturated fat by limiting the amount of fatty foods in your diet — particularly meats high in saturated fats like bacon, sausage, and prime rib. Stick to 1 or 2 servings per week and bake, broil, grill, stew, or stir-fry meats to reduce fat. Trim the fat off red meats and remove the skin from chicken before cooking.

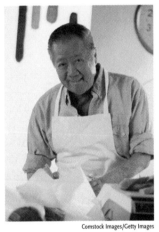

Comstock Images/Getty Images

Ask the butcher to trim the fat off meat.

Try fish as a healthy grilling option.

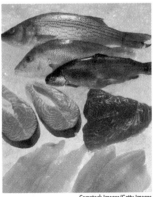

Comstock Images/Getty Images

Try not to become a man of success but rather try to become a man of value.
—Albert Einstein

Notes

MONDAY

Minutes of exercise _____
Weight _____
Blood pressure _____

TUESDAY

Minutes of exercise _____
Weight _____
Blood pressure _____

WEDNESDAY

Minutes of exercise _____
Weight _____
Blood pressure _____

THURSDAY

Minutes of exercise _____
Weight _____
Blood pressure _____

FRIDAY

Minutes of exercise _____
Weight _____
Blood pressure _____

SATURDAY

Minutes of exercise _____
Weight _____
Blood pressure _____

SUNDAY

Minutes of exercise _____
Weight _____
Blood pressure _____

Things to do for next week:

Check next week's supply of:
- blood pressure medication
- cholesterol medication
- aspirin
- vitamins
- diabetes medication
- lancets
- glucose test strips

Lemon and Herb Salmon Packets

PREP: 15 min GRILL: 14 min
4 servings

Ingredients
2 cups uncooked instant rice
1 can (14 ounces) fat-free or low-sodium chicken broth
1 cup matchstick-cut carrots (from 10-ounce bag)
4 salmon fillets (4 to 6 ounces each)
1 teaspoon lemon pepper seasoning salt
1/3 cup chopped fresh chives
1 medium lemon, cut lengthwise in half, then cut crosswise into 1/4-inch slices

1 Heat coals or gas grill for direct heat. Spray four 18 x 12-inch sheets of heavy-duty aluminum foil with cooking spray.

2 Mix rice and broth in medium bowl. Let stand about 5 minutes or until most of broth is absorbed. Stir in carrots.

3 Place salmon fillet on center of each foil sheet. Sprinkle with lemon pepper seasoning salt; top with chives. Arrange lemon slices over salmon. Spoon rice mixture around each fillet. Fold foil over salmon and rice so edges meet. Seal edges, making tight 1/2-inch fold; fold again. Allow space on sides for circulation and expansion.

4 Cover and grill packets 4 to 6 inches from low heat 11 to 14 minutes or until salmon flakes easily with fork. Place packets on plates. Cut large X across top of each packet; carefully fold back foil to allow steam to escape.

2.5 Carbohydrate Choices

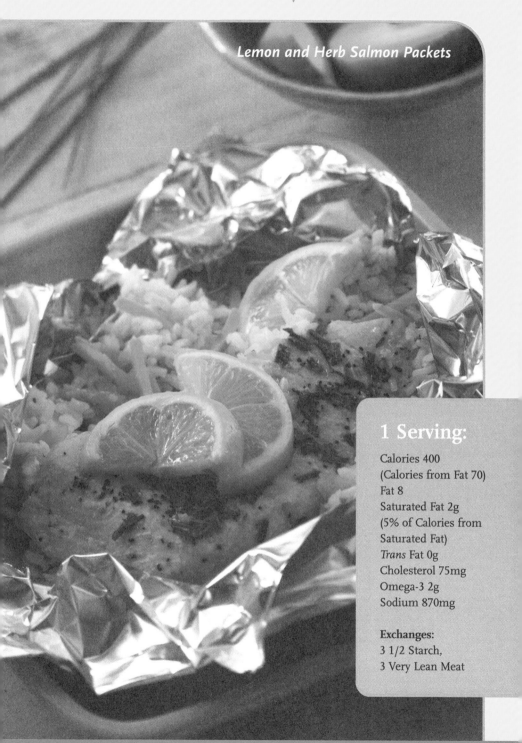

Lemon and Herb Salmon Packets

1 Serving:

Calories 400
(Calories from Fat 70)
Fat 8
Saturated Fat 2g
(5% of Calories from
Saturated Fat)
Trans Fat 0g
Cholesterol 75mg
Omega-3 2g
Sodium 870mg

Exchanges:
3 1/2 Starch,
3 Very Lean Meat

Dietary Fats

Not all fats are bad fats. Monounsaturated fats (olive oil, canola oil, peanut butter, and nuts) are "good" fats. Polyunsaturated fats (margarine made with corn or safflower oils and some nuts) are "acceptable" fats. Saturated fats (lard, butter, and cream cheese) are "bad" fats. Particularly bad are "trans" fats like partially hydrogenated vegetable oils found in many snack foods.

If you have high cholesterol and are at risk for cardiovascular disease, or if you have already had a cardiac event, you should contact a dietitian about reducing saturated fat intake. The dietitian will also review your intake of alcohol, caffeine, salt, and sugar — especially sugars found in "no fat" snack foods.

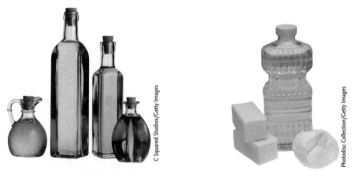

C Squared Studios/Getty Images

Photodisc Collection/Getty Images

Try to limit the amount of saturated fat in your diet.

The pessimist complains about the wind; the optimist expects the wind to change; the realist adjusts the sails.
—William Arthur Ward

Notes

MONDAY

Minutes of exercise _____
Weight _____
Blood pressure _____

TUESDAY

Minutes of exercise _____
Weight _____
Blood pressure _____

WEDNESDAY

Minutes of exercise _____
Weight _____
Blood pressure _____

THURSDAY

Minutes of exercise _____
Weight _____
Blood pressure _____

FRIDAY

Minutes of exercise _____
Weight _____
Blood pressure _____

SATURDAY

Minutes of exercise _____
Weight _____
Blood pressure _____

SUNDAY

Minutes of exercise _____
Weight _____
Blood pressure _____

Things to do for next week:

Check next week's supply of:
- ○ blood pressure medication
- ○ cholesterol medication
- ○ aspirin
- ○ vitamins
- ○ diabetes medication
- ○ lancets
- ○ glucose test strips

Bean and Barley Soup

PREP: 10 min COOK: 13 min
5 servings

Ingredients
1 tablespoon canola or soybean oil
2 small onions, sliced
2 cloves garlic, chopped
1 teaspoon ground cumin
1/2 cup uncooked quick-cooking barley
1 can (15 to 16 ounces) garbanzo beans, undrained
1 can (15 ounces) black beans, rinsed and drained
1 can (14 1/2 ounces) stewed tomatoes, undrained
1 package (10 ounces) frozen lima beans*
3 cups water
2 tablespoons chopped fresh cilantro or parsley

*1 can (15 to 16 ounces) lima beans, rinsed and drained, can be substituted
for the frozen lima beans.

1   Heat oil in 4-quart Dutch oven over medium heat. Cook
    onions, garlic and cumin in oil about 3 minutes, stirring
    occasionally, until onions are crisp-tender.

2   Stir in remaining ingredients
    except cilantro. Heat to boiling;
    reduce heat to low. Cover and
    simmer about 10 minutes or until
    lima beans are tender. Stir in
    cilantro.

1 Serving:

Calories 390
(Calories from Fat 55)
Fat 6g
Saturated Fat 1g
(1% of Calories from
Saturated Fat)
Trans Fat 0g
Cholesterol 0mg
Omega-3 0g
Sodium 940mg

Exchanges:
5 Starch, 1 Vegetable

5.5 Carbohydrate Choices

Barley, Corn and Lima Bean Sauté

PREP: 10 min COOK: 20 min STAND: 20 min
4 servings

Ingredients
1 1/3 cups water
2/3 cup uncooked quick-cooking barley
1 tablespoon butter
1 large onion, chopped (1 cup)
1 clove garlic, finely chopped
2 tablespoons chopped fresh or 2 teaspoons dried thyme leaves
1/2 teaspoon salt
1 bag (1 pound) frozen whole kernel corn, thawed and drained
1 package (10 ounces) frozen lima beans, thawed and drained

1 Heat water to boiling in 1 1/2-quart saucepan. Stir in barley; reduce heat to low. Cover and simmer 10 to 12 minutes or until tender. Let stand covered 5 minutes.

2 Melt butter in 10-inch skillet over medium-high heat. Cook onion and garlic in butter about 2 minutes, stirring occasionally, until onion is crisp-tender.

3 Stir in barley and remaining ingredients. Cook about 5 minutes, stirring occasionally, until thoroughly heated.

1 Serving:

Calories 335
(Calories from Fat 35)
Fat 4g
Saturated Fat 2g
(5% of Calories from
Saturated Fat)
Trans Fat 0g
Cholesterol 10mg
Omega-3 0g
Sodium 360mg

Exchanges:
4 Starch, 1 Other
Carbohydrates

5 Carbohydrate Choices

Calcium and Fat

To get the calcium you need without increasing your daily fat intake, try:

- Switching from whole milk to 1% or skim milk
- Using low-fat cheeses, yogurt, butter, and sour cream
- Eating low-fat ice cream or sherbet
- Drinking orange juice with added calcium

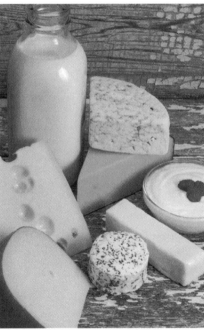

Comstock Images/Getty Images

Use low-fat cheese, yogurt, and milk to increase your calcium intake.

Notes

MONDAY

Minutes of exercise _____
Weight _____
Blood pressure _____

TUESDAY

Minutes of exercise _____
Weight _____
Blood pressure _____

WEDNESDAY

Minutes of exercise _____
Weight _____
Blood pressure _____

THURSDAY

Minutes of exercise _____
Weight _____
Blood pressure _____

FRIDAY

Minutes of exercise _____
Weight _____
Blood pressure _____

SATURDAY

Minutes of exercise _____
Weight _____
Blood pressure _____

SUNDAY

Minutes of exercise _____
Weight _____
Blood pressure _____

Things to do for next week:

Check next week's supply of:
- ○ blood pressure medication
- ○ cholesterol medication
- ○ aspirin
- ○ vitamins
- ○ diabetes medication
- ○ lancets
- ○ glucose test strips

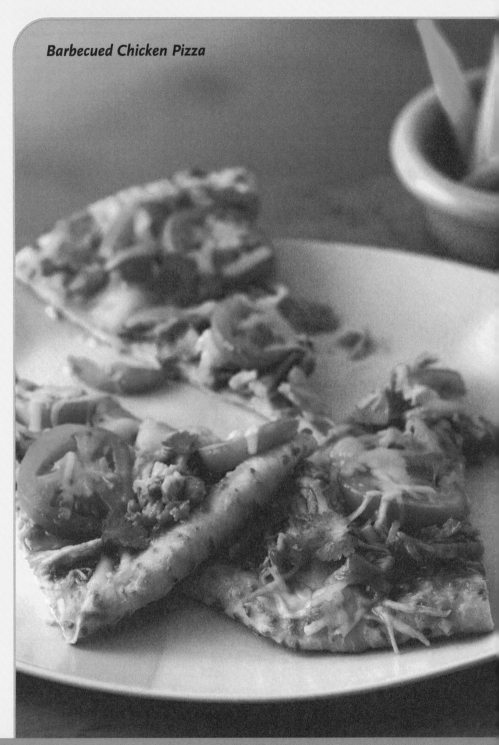

Barbecued Chicken Pizza

Barbecued Chicken Pizza

PREP: 10 min   BAKE: 10 min
6 servings

Ingredients
2 cups shredded cooked chicken breast
1/3 cup barbecue sauce
1 package (10 ounces) ready-to-serve thin Italian pizza crust (12 inches in
   diameter)
3 roma (plum) tomatoes, sliced
1 cup shredded reduced-fat Monterey Jack cheese (4 ounces)
Fresh cilantro leaves

1   Heat oven to 450°. Mix chicken and barbecue sauce in small
    bowl. Place pizza crust on ungreased cookie sheet; spread
    chicken mixture over crust. Arrange tomatoes over chicken;
    sprinkle with cheese.

2   Bake 10 minutes or until cheese is melted
    and crust is browned. Sprinkle with cilantro.

1 Serving:

Calories 285
(Calories from Fat 80)
Fat 9g
Saturated Fat 4g
(11% of Calories from
Saturated Fat)
Trans Fat 0g
Cholesterol 50mg
Omega-3 0g
Sodium 560mg

Exchanges:
2 Starch, 2 Lean Meat

2 Carbohydrate Choices

Food Journals

Keeping a journal of food intake can lead to weight loss. A food journal allows you to discover your meal plan's strengths and weaknesses and to identify areas for modification, if necessary. Follow these journaling tips:

- Record food intake after each meal when your memory is fresh.
- Log beverages as well as food.
- Be honest ... you want to identify your best cardiac-care practices.
- Measure foods to better understand portion sizes and to ensure accuracy.

Pages 277 to 279 of this journal provide space to complete a 3-day dietary recall. A registered dietitian can review the information and make recommendations for improving your diet.

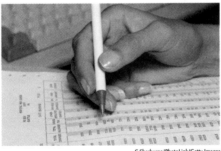

C Sherburne/PhotoLink/Getty Images

Talk to a registered dietitian about how to use a food journal to record your food consumption.

Motivation is what gets you started. Habit is what keeps you going.
—Jim Ryan

MONDAY

Minutes of exercise _____
Weight _____
Blood pressure _____

TUESDAY

Minutes of exercise _____
Weight _____
Blood pressure _____

WEDNESDAY

Minutes of exercise _____
Weight _____
Blood pressure _____

THURSDAY

Minutes of exercise _____
Weight _____
Blood pressure _____

FRIDAY

Minutes of exercise _____
Weight _____
Blood pressure _____

SATURDAY

Minutes of exercise _____
Weight _____
Blood pressure _____

SUNDAY

Minutes of exercise _____
Weight _____
Blood pressure _____

Things to do for next week:

Check next week's supply of:
- ○ blood pressure medication
- ○ cholesterol medication
- ○ aspirin
- ○ vitamins
- ○ diabetes medication
- ○ lancets
- ○ glucose test strips

Tuscan Panzanella Salad

PREP: 10 min
6 servings

Ingredients
1 bag (10 ounces) romaine and leaf lettuce mix
1 can (19 ounces) cannellini beans, rinsed and drained
2 cups large reduced-fat or fat-free croutons
1 cup sweet grape tomatoes
1/2 cup thinly sliced red onion
1/3 cup pitted Kalamata olives, cut in half
1/3 cup balsamic vinaigrette

1   Toss all ingredients except vinaigrette in large bowl.

2   Pour vinaigrette over salad; toss to coat.

1 Serving:

Calories 215
(Calories from Fat 65)
Fat 7g
Saturated Fat 1g
(3% of Calories from
Saturated Fat)
Trans Fat 0g
Cholesterol 0mg
Omega-3 0g
Sodium 270mg

Exchanges:
2 Starch, 1 Vegetable,
1 1/2 Lean Meat

2 Carbohydrate Choices

Saucy Raspberry-Rhubarb

PREP: 10 min COOK: 15 min COOL: 30 min
6 servings

Ingredients
3 cups chopped fresh rhubarb or 1 bag (16 ounces) frozen cut rhubarb,
  thawed
1/2 cup apple juice
3 tablespoons packed brown sugar
1 pint (2 cups) fresh raspberries
6 tablespoons reduced-fat sour cream

1   Heat rhubarb, apple juice, brown sugar and 1 cup of the
    raspberries to boiling in 1 1/2-quart saucepan; reduce heat.
    Simmer uncovered about 10 minutes, stirring occasionally,
    until rhubarb is soft. Cool about 30 minutes.

2   Stir in remaining 1 cup raspberries. Spoon into dessert
    dishes. Top with sour cream.

1 Serving:

Calories 85
(Calories from Fat 10)
Fat 1g
Saturated Fat 1g
(7% of Calories from
Saturated Fat)
Trans Fat 0g
Cholesterol 5mg
Omega-3 0g
Sodium 20mg

Exchanges:
1 Fruit

1 Carbohydrate Choice

The Good Egg

If you have a history of heart disease, elevated cholesterol, or diabetes, limit your intake of egg yolks to no more than 3 or 4 per week. Egg whites or "egg substitutes" have no cholesterol and do not need to be limited.

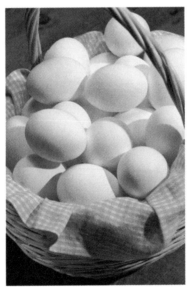

Limit the number of egg yolks to 3 or 4 per week.

Comstock Images/Getty Images

Notes

MONDAY

Minutes of exercise _____
Weight _____
Blood pressure _____

TUESDAY

Minutes of exercise _____
Weight _____
Blood pressure _____

WEDNESDAY

Minutes of exercise _____
Weight _____
Blood pressure _____

THURSDAY

Minutes of exercise _____
Weight _____
Blood pressure _____

FRIDAY

Minutes of exercise _____
Weight _____
Blood pressure _____

SATURDAY

Minutes of exercise _____
Weight _____
Blood pressure _____

SUNDAY

Minutes of exercise _____
Weight _____
Blood pressure _____

Things to do for next week:

Check next week's supply of:
○ blood pressure medication
○ cholesterol medication
○ aspirin
○ vitamins
○ diabetes medication
○ lancets
○ glucose test strips

Crème Caramel

PREP: 30 min   BAKE: 30 min   CHILL: 3 hr
8 servings

Ingredients

1 cup sugar
1 3/4 cups fat-free (skim) milk
1 cup fat-free cholesterol-free egg product
   or 8 egg whites
2 cups raspberries, blackberries, blueberries
   or sliced strawberries

1/4 teaspoon salt
1 teaspoon vanilla

1 Heat oven to 325°. Heat 1/2 cup of the sugar in medium
   nonstick skillet over medium heat 7 to 10 minutes, stirring
   frequently with wooden spoon, until sugar is melted and a
   light caramel color (mixture will be very hot and could melt a
   plastic spoon). Immediately pour sugar mixture into round
   pan, 8 x 1 1/2 inches; tilt pan to coat bottom. Place on wire
   rack to cool.

2 Mix remaining 1/2 cup sugar, milk, egg product, salt and
   vanilla in large bowl. Pour mixture over sugar mixture in pan.
   Place in rectangular pan 13 x 9 x 2 inches. Pour very hot water
   into rectangular pan to within
   1/2 inch of top of round pan.

3 Bake 50 to 60 minutes or until
   knife inserted in center comes out
   clean. Remove round pan from
   pan of water. Cover; refrigerate
   until thoroughly chilled, about
   3 hours or overnight. To unmold,
   run knife around edge of custard
   to loosen; invert onto serving
   platter. Top with fruit.

1 Serving:

Calories 150
(Calories from Fat 0)
Fat 0g
Saturated Fat 0g
(0% of Calories from
Saturated Fat)
Trans Fat 0g
Cholesterol 0mg
Omega-3 0g
Sodium 160mg

Exchanges:
1 Fruit, 1/2 Milk,
1 Other Carbohydrates

2 Carbohydrate Choices

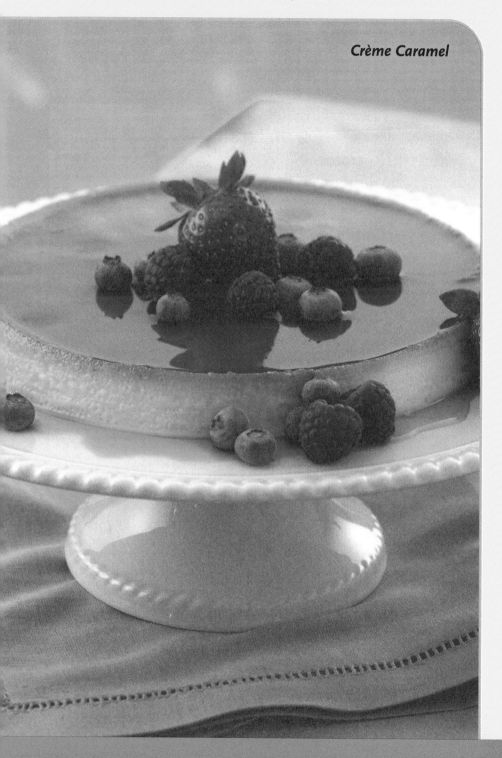

Crème Caramel

Fiber

Fiber — found in fruits, vegetables, beans, legumes, and whole grains — provides many health benefits to you, including:

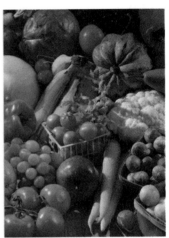

Comstock Images/Getty Images

- Soluble fiber (especially oats and barley) helps lower cholesterol levels
- Maintaining a healthy digestive tract
- Controlling weight by making you feel full to prevent overeating

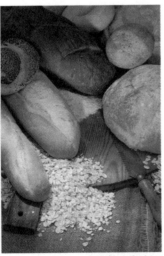

Comstock Images/Getty Images

Incorporate more fiber into your diet by:

- Adding dried fruits to salads
- Using oats (instead of bread crumbs) in meatloaf
- Adding berries to your cereal
- Replacing white rice and breads with brown rice and whole-grain breads
- Adding fresh vegetables to homemade pizza

Courage is doing what you're afraid to do. There can be no courage unless you're scared.
—Eddie Rickenbacker

Notes

MONDAY

Minutes of exercise _____
Weight _____
Blood pressure _____

TUESDAY

Minutes of exercise _____
Weight _____
Blood pressure _____

WEDNESDAY

Minutes of exercise _____
Weight _____
Blood pressure _____

THURSDAY

Minutes of exercise _____
Weight _____
Blood pressure _____

FRIDAY

Minutes of exercise _____
Weight _____
Blood pressure _____

SATURDAY

Minutes of exercise _____
Weight _____
Blood pressure _____

SUNDAY

Minutes of exercise _____
Weight _____
Blood pressure _____

Things to do for next week:

Check next week's supply of:
- ○ blood pressure medication
- ○ cholesterol medication
- ○ aspirin
- ○ vitamins
- ○ diabetes medication
- ○ lancets
- ○ glucose test strips

Oatmeal Pancakes

PREP: 10 min COOK: 15 min
4 servings (9 pancakes)

Ingredients
1/2 cup quick-cooking or old-fashioned oats
1/4 cup all-purpose flour
1/4 cup whole wheat flour
1 tablespoon sugar
1 teaspoon baking powder
1/2 teaspoon baking soda
1/2 teaspoon salt
3/4 cup buttermilk
1/4 cup fat-free (skim) milk
1/4 cup fat-free cholesterol-free egg product, thawed or 2 egg whites
2 tablespoons canola or soybean oil

1   Beat all ingredients in large bowl with hand beater or wire whisk just until smooth. (For thinner pancakes, stir in additional 2 to 4 tablespoons milk.)

2   Spray griddle or 10-inch nonstick skillet with cooking spray; heat griddle to 375° or skillet over medium heat. (To test griddle, sprinkle with a few drops of water. If bubbles skitter around, heat is just right.)

3   For each pancake, pour slightly less than 1/4 cup batter onto hot griddle. Cook pancakes until puffed and dry around edges. Turn; cook other sides until golden brown.

1 Serving:

Calories 200
(Calories from Fat 70)
Fat 8g
Saturated Fat 1g
(4% of Calories from
Saturated Fat)
Trans Fat 0g
Cholesterol 0mg
Omega-3 0g
Sodium 660mg

Exchanges:
1 1/2 Starch,
1 1/2 Fat

1.5 Carbohydrate Choices

Hot Crab-Artichoke Dip

PREP: 15 min BAKE: 25 min
15 servings (2 tablespoons dip and 4 crackers)

Ingredients
1/3 cup plain fat-free yogurt
3 tablespoons reduced-fat mayonnaise
1/4 cup grated Parmesan cheese
2 cloves garlic, finely chopped
6 ounces imitation crabmeat, chopped
1 can (14 ounces) artichoke hearts, drained and coarsely chopped
1 can (4 1/2 ounces) chopped green chiles, drained
Dash of paprika
60 water crackers

1 Heat oven to 350˚. Spray 1-quart casserole with cooking spray. Mix yogurt, mayonnaise, cheese and garlic in medium bowl. Stir in crabmeat, artichoke hearts and chiles. Spoon into casserole.

2 Bake uncovered about 25 minutes or until golden brown and bubbly. Sprinkle with paprika before serving. Serve with crackers.

1 Serving:

Calories 95
(Calories from Fat 20)
Fat 2g
Saturated Fat 1g
(6% of Calories from Saturated Fat)
Trans Fat 0g
Cholesterol 5mg
Omega-3 0g
Sodium 320mg

Exchanges:
1 Starch,
1/2 Very Lean Meat

1 Carbohydrate Choice

Let's See Where You Are

If you have been using this journal faithfully each week, you should be about halfway through the year. Let's stop and see how you are doing.

1) Have you had your blood tests done? Be sure that your doctor measures your cholesterol, blood sugar (blood glucose), and liver function (if you take a statin medication). Keep a record of your test results in the back of this journal (see page 282).

2) Have you seen the members of your healthcare team at least according to the following yearly schedule:

- Family doctor 3 times
- Cardiologist 2 times
- Registered dietitian 1 time

3) Have you been refilling your medications on time? Be sure to make a note in your journal when your next refill is due.

Even if you're on the right track, you'll get run over if you just sit there.
—Will Rogers

Notes

MONDAY

Minutes of exercise _____
Weight _____
Blood pressure _____

TUESDAY

Minutes of exercise _____
Weight _____
Blood pressure _____

WEDNESDAY

Minutes of exercise _____
Weight _____
Blood pressure _____

THURSDAY

Minutes of exercise _____
Weight _____
Blood pressure _____

FRIDAY

Minutes of exercise _____
Weight _____
Blood pressure _____

SATURDAY

Minutes of exercise _____
Weight _____
Blood pressure _____

SUNDAY

Minutes of exercise _____
Weight _____
Blood pressure _____

Things to do for next week:

Check next week's supply of:
- ○ blood pressure medication
- ○ cholesterol medication
- ○ aspirin
- ○ vitamins
- ○ diabetes medication
- ○ lancets
- ○ glucose test strips

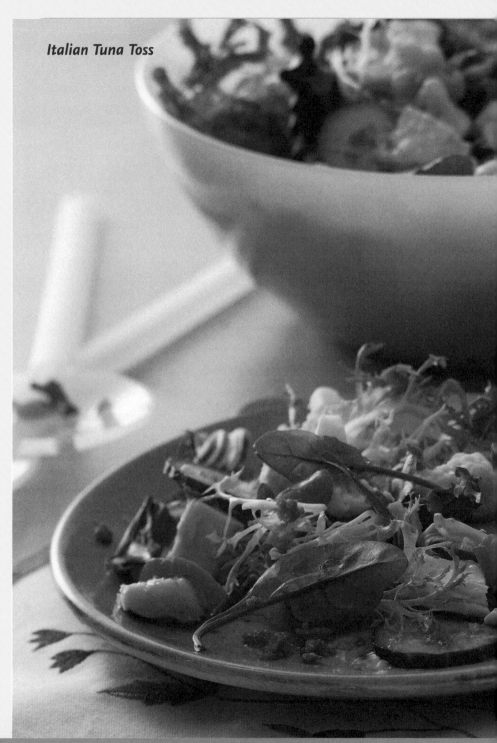

Italian Tuna Toss

Italian Tuna Toss

PREP: 10 min
6 servings

Ingredients
1 medium cucumber, sliced (1 1/2 cups)
2 cans (6 ounces each) tuna in water, drained
1 bag (16 ounces) fresh cauliflower florets
1 bag (10 ounces) mixed salad greens
1 jar (2 ounces) sliced pimientos, drained (1/4 cup)
1/3 cup Italian dressing
1/4 cup bacon flavor bits or chips

1   Toss all ingredients except dressing and bacon bits in large
    bowl.

2   Pour dressing over salad and sprinkle with bacon bits; toss
    to mix.

1 Serving:

Calories 170
(Calories from Fat 65)
Fat 7g
Saturated Fat 1g
(4% of Calories from
Saturated Fat)
Trans Fat 0g
Cholesterol 20mg
Omega-3 0g
Sodium 400mg

Exchanges:
2 Vegetable, 2 Lean Meat

2.5 Carbohydrate Choices

Alcohol Consumption

Excessive alcohol consumption over time can lead to many harmful effects, including high blood pressure, cirrhosis of the liver, and damage to the heart. Women should not consume more than 1 drink per day — 5 ounces of wine, 12 ounces of beer, or 1-1/2 ounces of 80-proof liquor. Men should not consume more than 2 drinks daily.

The following individuals should not drink alcohol at all:

- People with high levels of triglycerides in their blood (over 300 mg/dL)
- Pregnant women
- Those who are under the legal drinking age
- People with a genetic predisposition for alcoholism or who are recovering from alcoholism
- People taking certain medications (ask your doctor or pharmacist)

Talk to your doctor about heart disease and alcohol consumption.

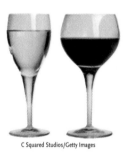

C Squared Studios/Getty Images

So many tangles in life are so ultimately hopeless we have no appropriate sword other than laughter.
—George W. Allport

MONDAY

Minutes of exercise _____
Weight _____
Blood pressure _____

TUESDAY

Minutes of exercise _____
Weight _____
Blood pressure _____

WEDNESDAY

Minutes of exercise _____
Weight _____
Blood pressure _____

THURSDAY

Minutes of exercise _____
Weight _____
Blood pressure _____

FRIDAY

Minutes of exercise _____
Weight _____
Blood pressure _____

SATURDAY

Minutes of exercise _____
Weight _____
Blood pressure _____

SUNDAY

Minutes of exercise _____
Weight _____
Blood pressure _____

Things to do for next week:

Check next week's supply of:

- ○ blood pressure medication
- ○ cholesterol medication
- ○ aspirin
- ○ vitamins
- ○ diabetes medication
- ○ lancets
- ○ glucose test strips

Pecan-Crusted Catfish

PREP: 10 min BAKE: 20 min
4 servings

Ingredients
1/2 cup cornflake crumbs
1/4 cup finely ground pecans (1 ounce)
1/4 teaspoon paprika
1/8 teaspoon garlic powder
1/8 teaspoon ground red pepper (cayenne)
1 egg white
1 pound catfish, haddock, orange roughy, sole, flounder or other
  medium-firm fish fillets, about 3/4 inch thick, cut into 4 pieces

1   Heat oven to 450°. Spray jelly roll pan, 15 1/2 x 10 1/2 x 1 inch,
    with cooking spray. Mix cornflake crumbs, pecans, paprika,
    garlic powder and ground red pepper in large resealable
    plastic food-storage bag.

2   Beat egg white slightly with fork in shallow dish. Dip fish into
    egg white, then place in bag. Seal bag and shake until evenly
    coated. Place in pan.

3   Bake 15 to 20 minutes or until fish
    flakes easily with fork.

1 Serving:

Calories 225
(Calories from Fat 110)
Fat 12g
Saturated Fat 2g
(7% of Calories from
Saturated Fat)
Trans Fat 0g
Cholesterol 85mg
Omega-3 1g
Sodium 105mg

Exchanges:
1/2 Fat, 3 1/2 Lean Meat

0 Carbohydrate Choices

Turkey–Wild Rice Soup

PREP: 10 min COOK: 26 min
10 servings

Ingredients
1 tablespoon butter
2 tablespoons canola or soybean oil
1/2 cup all-purpose flour
2 cups water
2 cups cut-up cooked turkey, chicken or ham
2 cans (14 ounces each) chicken broth
1 jar (4 1/2 ounces) sliced mushrooms, drained
2 tablespoons instant chopped onion
1 package (6 ounces) original-flavor long-grain and wild rice mix
2 cups original soy milk or fat-free (skim) milk
1/4 cup slivered almonds, toasted*

*To toast nuts, bake uncovered in ungreased shallow pan in 350° oven about 10 minutes, stirring occasionally, until golden brown. Or cook in ungreased heavy skillet over medium-low heat 5 to 7 minutes, stirring frequently until browning begins, then stirring constantly until golden brown.

1 Melt butter in 5-quart Dutch oven over medium heat. Stir in oil and flour with wire whisk until well blended. Stir in water, turkey, broth, mushrooms, onion, rice and rice seasoning packet.

2 Heat to boiling over high heat, stirring occasionally. Reduce heat to medium-low. Cover and simmer about 25 minutes or until rice is tender.

3 Stir in soy milk; heat just to boiling. Remove from heat. Sprinkle each serving with almonds.

1 Serving:

Calories 190
(Calories from Fat 80)
Fat 9g
Saturated Fat 2g
(9% of Calories from
Saturated Fat)
Trans Fat 0g
Cholesterol 25mg
Omega-3 0g
Sodium 480mg

Exchanges:
1 Starch,
1 1/2 Medium-Fat Meat

1 Carbohydrate Choice

Eating Right

A healthy diet is crucial part of your overall health. Because one diet does not work for everyone, you should meet with a registered dietitian to set up your own meal plan. After reviewing your lab results and lifestyle, the dietitian will discuss treatment options. The diet is a form of treatment — medical nutrition therapy — designed just for you.

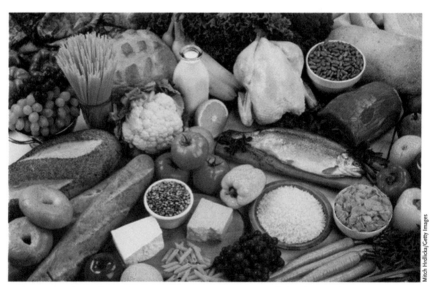

Meet with a dietitian to set up a well-balanced diet.

I'm a self-made man. But I think if I had it to do over again, I'd call in someone else.
—Roland Young

Notes

MONDAY

Minutes of exercise _____
Weight _____
Blood pressure _____

TUESDAY

Minutes of exercise _____
Weight _____
Blood pressure _____

WEDNESDAY

Minutes of exercise _____
Weight _____
Blood pressure _____

THURSDAY

Minutes of exercise _____
Weight _____
Blood pressure _____

FRIDAY

Minutes of exercise _____
Weight _____
Blood pressure _____

SATURDAY

Minutes of exercise _____
Weight _____
Blood pressure _____

SUNDAY

Minutes of exercise _____
Weight _____
Blood pressure _____

Things to do for next week:

Check next week's supply of:

○ blood pressure medication
○ cholesterol medication
○ aspirin
○ vitamins
○ diabetes medication
○ lancets
○ glucose test strips

Southwestern Chicken BLT Salad

PREP: 20 min
6 servings

Ingredients
Salsa-Bacon Dressing (below)
1 bag (10 ounces) romaine and leaf lettuce mix
4 roma (plum) tomatoes, coarsely chopped
1/2 cup chopped cooked bacon
1/2 cup croutons
2 packages (6 ounces each) refrigerated cooked Southwest-flavor chicken
   breast strips

1 Make Salsa-Bacon Dressing; set aside.

2 Mix remaining ingredients in large bowl. Add dressing; toss
   until coated.

Salsa-Bacon Dressing
1/2 cup chunky-style salsa
1/2 cup nonfat ranch dressing
1 tablespoon chopped fresh parsley

   Mix all ingredients in small bowl.

1 Serving:

Calories 190
(Calories from Fat 44)
Fat 6g
Saturated Fat 2g
(9% calories from
Saturated Fat)
Trans Fat 0g
Cholesterol 55mg
Omega-3 0g
Sodium 580mg

Exchanges:
1/2 Starch, 1 Vegetable,
3 Very Lean Meat,
1/2 Fat

2.5 Carbohydrate Choices

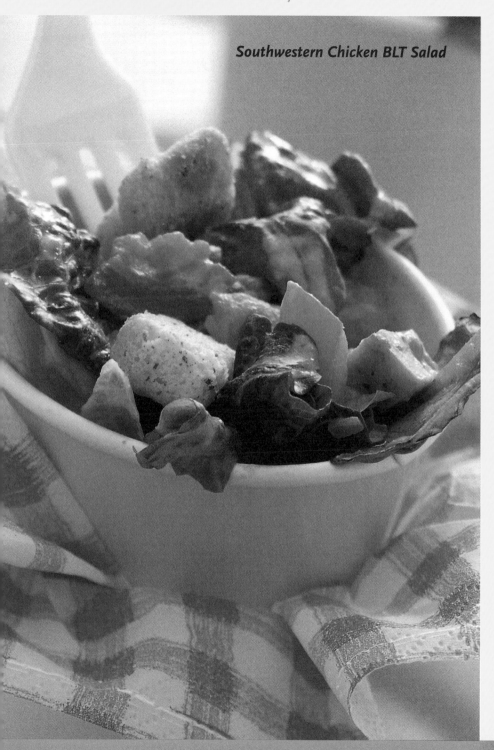

Southwestern Chicken BLT Salad

Common Medications

Medicines are used to prevent or control heart disease. Common medicines include anticoagulants ("blood thinners"), antiplatelet medicines, ACE or Angiotensin Receptor inhibitors, beta-blockers, calcium channel blockers, cholesterol-lowering medicines, digitalis, diuretics, and nitrates. Many of these medicines are used for more than one condition. For example, beta-blockers and calcium channel blockers are used for angina, high blood pressure and arrhythmia.

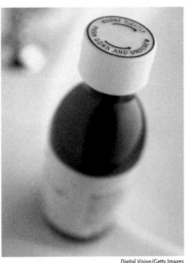

Digital Vision/Getty Images

If you have questions about your medications, be sure to discuss them with your doctor or pharmacist.

Notes

MONDAY

Minutes of exercise _____
Weight _____
Blood pressure _____

TUESDAY

Minutes of exercise _____
Weight _____
Blood pressure _____

WEDNESDAY

Minutes of exercise _____
Weight _____
Blood pressure _____

THURSDAY

Minutes of exercise _____
Weight _____
Blood pressure _____

FRIDAY

Minutes of exercise _____
Weight _____
Blood pressure _____

SATURDAY

Minutes of exercise _____
Weight _____
Blood pressure _____

SUNDAY

Minutes of exercise _____
Weight _____
Blood pressure _____

Things to do for next week:

Check next week's supply of:
○ blood pressure medication
○ cholesterol medication
○ aspirin
○ vitamins
○ diabetes medication
○ lancets
○ glucose test strips

Broccoli-Cheese Soup

PREP: 10 min COOK: 13 min
6 servings (1 cup each)

Ingredients
1 tablespoon canola or soybean oil
1 medium onion, chopped (1/2 cup)
1 tablespoon all-purpose flour
1 teaspoon salt
3 cups soy milk or fat-free (skim) milk
2 teaspoons cornstarch
1 1/2 cups shredded reduced-fat sharp Cheddar cheese (6 ounces)
3 cups bite-size fresh or frozen (thawed) broccoli flowerets
1 cup low-fat popped popcorn, if desired

1   Heat oil in 3-quart saucepan over medium heat. Stir in onion, flour and salt. Cook 2 to 3 minutes, stirring constantly, until onion is soft.

2   Stir soy milk and cornstarch in small bowl with wire whisk until smooth. Gradually stir into onion mixture. Cook 5 to 6 minutes, stirring frequently, until thick and bubbly.

3   Stir in cheese. Cook about 3 minutes, stirring frequently, until cheese is melted. Stir in broccoli. Cook about 1 minute or until hot, stirring occasionally. If desired, top this creamy cheese soup with popcorn.

1 Serving:

Calories 140
(Calories from Fat 45)
Fat 5g
Saturated Fat 1g
(10% of Calories from
Saturated Fat)
Trans Fat 0g
Cholesterol 5mg
Omega-3 0g
Sodium 730mg

Exchanges:
1/2 Milk, 1 Vegetable,
1/2 Fat, 1/2 High-Fat
Meat

1 Carbohydrate Choice

Roasted Sweet Pepper Pasta Salad with Herbs and Feta

PREP: 10 min BAKE: 20 min COOK: 10 min
6 servings

Ingredients
2 large red or yellow bell peppers, cut into 1-inch pieces
1 medium red onion, cut into wedges (about 2 cups)
Cooking spray
3 cups uncooked penne pasta (10 ounces)
1 cup sliced 70%-less-fat turkey pepperoni (about 3 ounces), cut in half
2 ounces feta cheese, crumbled (1/2 cup)
1/2 cup fat-free Italian dressing
2 tablespoons chopped fresh basil leaves
1 tablespoon chopped fresh mint leaves

1 Heat oven to 450°. Spray rectangular pan, 13 x 9 x 2 inches, with cooking spray. Place bell peppers and onion in single layer in pan. Spray vegetables with cooking spray. Bake uncovered 15 to 20 minutes or until vegetables are lightly browned and tender.

2 Meanwhile, cook and drain pasta as directed on package. Rinse with cold water; drain.

3 Toss bell peppers, onion, pasta and remaining ingredients in large bowl. Serve immediately, or refrigerate 1 to 2 hours.

1 Serving:

Calories 270
(Calories from Fat 45)
Fat 5g
Saturated Fat 2g
(7% of Calories from Saturated Fat)
Trans Fat 0g
Cholesterol 20mg
Omega-3 0g
Sodium 640mg

Exchanges:
2 1/2 Starch, 1 Vegetable, 1 Lean Meat

3 **Carbohydrate Choices**

Warm-up and Cooldown

Start with a warm-up before exercise (several minutes of easy walking) and end with a cooldown after exercise (again, several minutes of easy walking). Ask an exercise specialist for some recommendations for stretching after your workout, and discuss the intensity of the exercise with your doctor. If you feel any chest discomfort, discontinue your exercise and consult your doctor.

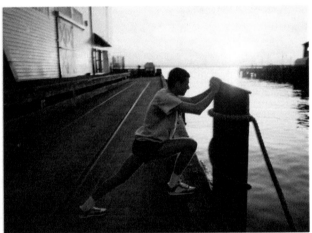

Photolink/Getty Images

Be sure to warm up prior to exercise and cool down afterward.

As a child my family's menu consisted of two choices: take it or leave it.
—Buddy Hackett

Notes

MONDAY

Minutes of exercise _____
Weight _____
Blood pressure _____

TUESDAY

Minutes of exercise _____
Weight _____
Blood pressure _____

WEDNESDAY

Minutes of exercise _____
Weight _____
Blood pressure _____

THURSDAY

Minutes of exercise _____
Weight _____
Blood pressure _____

FRIDAY

Minutes of exercise _____
Weight _____
Blood pressure _____

SATURDAY

Minutes of exercise _____
Weight _____
Blood pressure _____

SUNDAY

Minutes of exercise _____
Weight _____
Blood pressure _____

Things to do for next week:

Check next week's supply of:
○ blood pressure medication
○ cholesterol medication
○ aspirin
○ vitamins
○ diabetes medication
○ lancets
○ glucose test strips

Peach Melba Pancakes

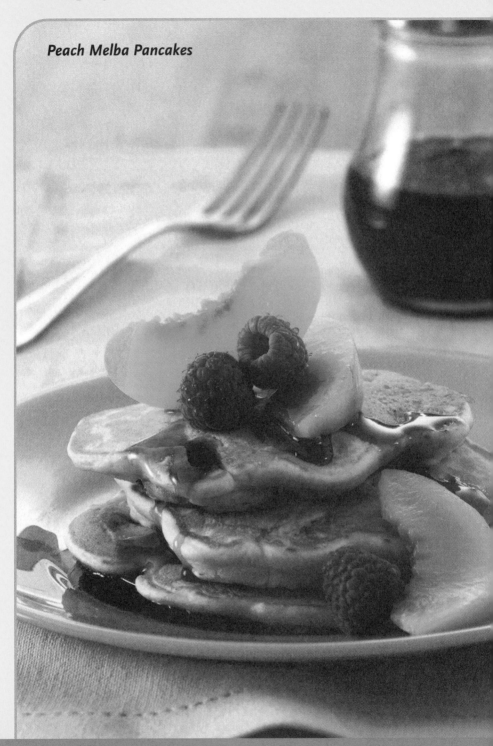

Peach Melba Pancakes

PREP: 10 min COOK: 15 min
9 servings (18 four-inch pancakes)

Ingredients
2 eggs
2 tablespoons sugar
2 cups all-purpose flour
1/2 teaspoon salt
3 teaspoons baking powder
1 1/2 cups milk
1/4 cup canola or soybean oil
1/2 cup chopped canned (drained) or frozen (thawed and drained) sliced
  peaches
1/2 cup fresh or frozen (thawed and well drained) raspberries
Additional peaches and raspberries, if desired
Raspberry syrup, if desired

1 Heat griddle to 375° or heat 10-inch skillet over medium heat; grease with shortening if necessary (or spray with cooking spray before heating).

2 Beat eggs in medium bowl with wire whisk until well beaten. Beat in flour, sugar, baking powder, salt, milk and oil just until smooth. Stir in 1/2 cup each peaches and raspberries.

3 For each pancake, pour slightly less than 1/4 cup batter onto hot griddle. Cook pancakes until bubbly on top, puffed and dry around edges. Turn; cook other sides until golden brown. Serve with additional peaches and raspberries and syrup.

1 Serving:

Calories 205
(Calories from Fat 70)
Fat 8g
Saturated Fat 1g
(4% of Calories from
Saturated Fat)
Trans Fat 0g
Cholesterol 45mg
Omega-3 0g
Sodium 330mg

Exchanges:
2 Starch, 1 Fat

3 Carbohydrate Choices

Healthy Snacks

Everyone enjoys an occasional snack. Eating small, frequent meals or snacks (every 4 to 5 hours) can help keep blood-sugar levels regulated. It may be beneficial, especially if you are taking insulin, to eat a small snack one-half to 1 hour prior to going to bed. Here are some ideas for tasty, yet healthy, snacks:

- 3 cups air-popped popcorn with fat-free liquid butter and 1 teaspoon of Parmesan cheese
- 1 cup baked tortilla chips and 2-3 tablespoons salsa
- 6 crackers with 1 ounce of string cheese or 1 ounce of 2% milk cheese
- 1 1/2 ounces of pretzels and 1 tablespoon natural peanut butter
- Raw veggies and low-fat veggie dip
- 3 graham crackers and 1 cup 1% milk
- 2-ounce slice of angel food cake with fresh berries
- Half a bagel with tomato sauce and low-fat cheese
- 1 cup sugar-free yogurt with 2 tablespoons of granola
- Apple or banana with 1 to 2 tablespoons natural peanut butter

Enjoy!

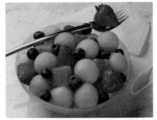

Mitch Hrdlicka/Getty Images

Try a medley of fruits as a healthy snack.

Notes

MONDAY

Minutes of exercise _____
Weight _____
Blood pressure _____

TUESDAY

Minutes of exercise _____
Weight _____
Blood pressure _____

WEDNESDAY

Minutes of exercise _____
Weight _____
Blood pressure _____

THURSDAY

Minutes of exercise _____
Weight _____
Blood pressure _____

FRIDAY

Minutes of exercise _____
Weight _____
Blood pressure _____

SATURDAY

Minutes of exercise _____
Weight _____
Blood pressure _____

SUNDAY

Minutes of exercise _____
Weight _____
Blood pressure _____

Things to do for next week:

Check next week's supply of:
- ○ blood pressure medication
- ○ cholesterol medication
- ○ aspirin
- ○ vitamins
- ○ diabetes medication
- ○ lancets
- ○ glucose test strips

Caribbean Crabmeat Pasta Salad

PREP: 10 min
6 servings

Ingredients
3 cups uncooked rotelle pasta (8 ounces)
Honey-Lime Dressing (below)
1 package (8 ounces) refrigerated flake-style imitation crabmeat
1 medium red bell pepper, cut into thin bite-size strips
1 medium mango, peeled, seeded and cubed (about 1 cup)
1/2 to 1 jalapeño chili, seeded and finely chopped
2 tablespoons chopped fresh cilantro

1   Cook and drain pasta as directed on package. Rinse with cold water; drain.

2   Meanwhile, make Honey-Lime Dressing.

3   Gently toss pasta and remaining ingredients in large bowl. Pour dressing over salad; toss gently to coat. Cover and refrigerate at least 1 hour to blend flavors.

Honey-Lime Dressing
1 teaspoon grated lime peel
3 tablespoons lime juice
2 tablespoons canola or soybean oil
1 tablespoon honey
1/2 teaspoon ground cumin
1/2 teaspoon ground ginger
1/4 teaspoon salt

Mix all ingredients in small bowl until well blended.

1 Serving:

Calories 270
(Calories from Fat 55)
Fat 6g
Saturated Fat 1g
(2% of Calories from
Saturated Fat)
Trans Fat 0g
Cholesterol 10mg
Omega-3 0g
Sodium 430mg

Exchanges: 2 Starch,
1 Fruit, 1 Very Lean Meat,
1/2 Fat

3 Carbohydrate Choices

Frosty Margarita Pie

PREP: 15 min FREEZE: 1 hr 30 min
6 servings (1 cup each)

Ingredients
3/4 cup graham cracker crumbs (10 squares)
1/2 cup finely chopped strawberries
1/2 cup sugar
1 quart (4 cups) vanilla fat-free frozen yogurt
1 tablespoon grated lime peel
1/3 cup lime juice
2 to 4 tablespoons tequila, if desired
1 cup frozen (thawed) reduced-fat whipped topping, if desired
Lime and strawberry slices, if desired

1   Mix cracker crumbs, chopped strawberries and sugar in small bowl. Press in bottom and up sides of pie plate, 9 x 1 1/4 inches; set aside.

2   Beat yogurt, lime peel, lime juice and tequila in large bowl with electric mixer on high speed just until blended. Spoon into crust. Freeze at least 1 1/2 hours or until firm enough to cut. Serve topped with whipped topping; garnish with lime and strawberry slices.

1 Serving:

Calories 195
(Calories from Fat 10)
Fat 1g
Saturated Fat 0g
(1% of Calories from Saturated Fat)
Trans Fat 0g
Cholesterol 0mg
Omega-3 0g
Sodium 95mg

Exchanges:
1 Starch, 2 Other Carbohydrates

3 Carbohydrate Choices

Childhood Obesity

Obesity is very closely related to the development and progression of diabetes.

Obesity results from an imbalance in the number of calories consumed (eating too much) versus calories expended (not exercising enough), causing the body to store extra fat. This often leads to a condition called "insulin resistance" that may eventually develop into type 2 diabetes.

Children who are obese should reduce their weight with diet and exercise. Exercise helps by burning calories, and it also enables the muscle cells to use insulin more effectively.

Notes

MONDAY

Minutes of exercise _____
Weight _____
Blood pressure _____

TUESDAY

Minutes of exercise _____
Weight _____
Blood pressure _____

WEDNESDAY

Minutes of exercise _____
Weight _____
Blood pressure _____

THURSDAY

Minutes of exercise _____
Weight _____
Blood pressure _____

FRIDAY

Minutes of exercise _____
Weight _____
Blood pressure _____

SATURDAY

Minutes of exercise _____
Weight _____
Blood pressure _____

SUNDAY

Minutes of exercise _____
Weight _____
Blood pressure _____

Things to do for next week:

Check next week's supply of:
- ○ blood pressure medication
- ○ cholesterol medication
- ○ aspirin
- ○ vitamins
- ○ diabetes medication
- ○ lancets
- ○ glucose test strips

Mocha Cappuccino Pudding Cake

PREP: 10 min BAKE: 45 min
12 servings

Ingredients
1 1/4 cups all-purpose flour
1 3/4 cups sugar
1/4 cup baking cocoa
1 tablespoon instant espresso coffee (dry)
1 1/2 teaspoons baking powder
1/2 teaspoon salt
1/2 cup fat-free (skim) milk
2 tablespoons butter, melted or canola or soybean oil
1 teaspoon vanilla
1 teaspoon instant espresso coffee (dry)
1 1/2 cups very warm fat-free (skim) milk (120° to 130°)

1 Heat oven to 350°. Mix flour, 3/4 cup of the sugar, 2 tablespoons of the cocoa, 1 tablespoon espresso coffee, the baking powder and salt in medium bowl. Stir in 1/2 cup milk, butter and vanilla until well blended. Spread in ungreased square pan, 9 x 9 x 2 inches.

2 Mix remaining 1 cup sugar, remaining 2 tablespoons cocoa and 1 teaspoon espresso coffee in small bowl; sprinkle evenly over cake batter. Pour 1 1/2 cups very warm milk over sugar mixture.

3 Bake 35 to 45 minutes or until center is set and firm to the touch. Place sheet of aluminum foil or cookie sheet on lower oven rack under cake to catch any spills. Spoon warm cake into dessert dishes.

1 Serving:

Calories 205
(Calories from Fat 20)
Fat 2g
Saturated Fat 1g
(6% of Calories from
Saturated Fat)
Trans Fat 0g
Cholesterol 5mg
Omega-3 0g
Sodium 190mg

Exchanges:
1/2 Milk, 2 1/2 Other
Carbohydrates

3 Carbohydrate Choices

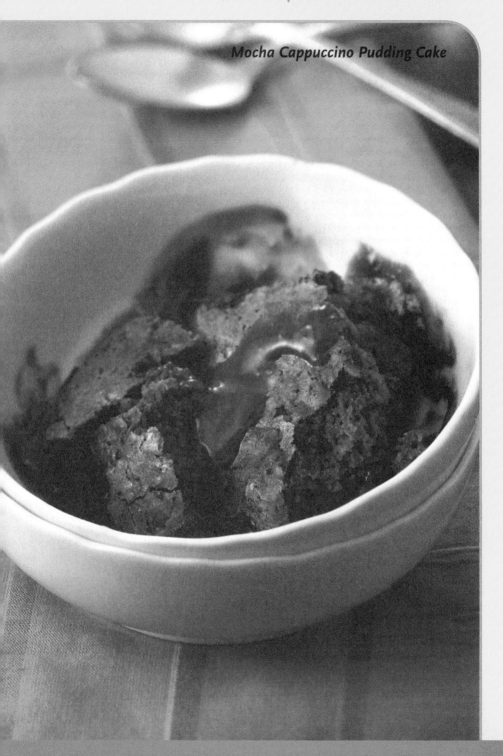

Mocha Cappuccino Pudding Cake

Obese vs. Overweight

People who are 20% over the recommended weight for their height (according to Metropolitan Life's height/weight tables) are considered to be overweight — but not necessarily obese. Obesity refers to "fatness" rather than weight. Men who have more than 25% of their body weight as fat and women who have more than 35% are "obese."

Central obesity (indicated by an apple-shaped body) is closely related to diabetes and heart disease. You might have central obesity if your waist girth measures more than 35 inches (for females) or more than 40 inches (for males).

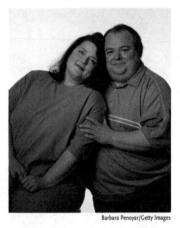

Barbara Penoyar/Getty Images

Talk to a registered dietitian about how to modify your diet to help you begin a weight-loss program.

There are too many people praying for mountains of difficulty to be removed, when what they really need is courage to climb them.   —Unknown

Notes

MONDAY

Minutes of exercise _____
Weight _____
Blood pressure _____

TUESDAY

Minutes of exercise _____
Weight _____
Blood pressure _____

WEDNESDAY

Minutes of exercise _____
Weight _____
Blood pressure _____

THURSDAY

Minutes of exercise _____
Weight _____
Blood pressure _____

FRIDAY

Minutes of exercise _____
Weight _____
Blood pressure _____

SATURDAY

Minutes of exercise _____
Weight _____
Blood pressure _____

SUNDAY

Minutes of exercise _____
Weight _____
Blood pressure _____

Things to do for next week:

Check next week's supply of:
- ○ blood pressure medication
- ○ cholesterol medication
- ○ aspirin
- ○ vitamins
- ○ diabetes medication
- ○ lancets
- ○ glucose test strips

Rise-and-Shine Waffles

PREP: 10 min   BAKE: 5 min per waffle
8 servings

Ingredients

3/4 cup old-fashioned oats
1/4 cup packed brown sugar
1/4 teaspoon baking soda
Maple-Yogurt Topping (below)
3 tablespoons canola or soybean oil
2 tablespoons wheat germ or ground flax
1/4 cup fat-free cholesterol-free egg product, thawed or 2 egg whites, slightly beaten

2/3 cup all-purpose flour
2 teaspoons baking powder
1 cup fat-free (skim) milk
1 teaspoon grated orange peel

1 Mix oats, brown sugar and milk in large bowl; let stand 10 minutes. Meanwhile, make Maple-Yogurt Topping; set aside. Spray nonstick waffle iron with cooking spray; heat waffle iron.

2 Stir egg product and oil into oat mixture. Stir in remaining ingredients until blended.

3 For each waffle, pour 1 cup batter onto center of hot waffle iron; close lid. Bake 4 to 5 minutes or until steaming stops and waffle is golden brown. Carefully remove waffle. Serve with topping. Garnish with additional grated fresh orange peel and chopped cranberries, if desired.

Maple-Yogurt Topping
1 cup plain nonfat yogurt
1/4 cup maple syrup

Mix all ingredients until well blended.

1 Serving:

Calories 200
(Calories from Fat 55)
Fat 6g
Saturated Fat 1g
(3% of Calories from Saturated Fat)
Trans Fat 0g
Cholesterol 0mg
Omega-3 1g
Sodium 220mg

Exchanges:
2 Starch, 1 Fat

2 **Carbohydrate Choices**

Hiker's Trail Mix

PREP: 5 min
12 servings (1/2 cup each)

Ingredients
1 1/2 cups roasted soy nuts
1 cup Multigrain or Honey Nut Cheerios® cereal
3/4 cup raisins
1/2 cup candy-coated chocolate candies or chocolate chips

Mix all ingredients. Store in resealable plastic bag or tightly covered container.

1 Serving:

Calories 145
(Calories from Fat 45)
Fat 5g
Saturated Fat 2g
(11% of Calories from
Saturated Fat)
Trans Fat 0g
Cholesterol 0mg
Omega-3 0g
Sodium 40mg

Exchanges:
1 Starch, 1 Fat, 1/2 Other
Carbohydrates

1 Carbohydrate Choice

Traveling and Heart Disease

Before leaving, notify your doctor of travel plans and get a complete physical exam to be sure your heart condition is well controlled.

When traveling, be sure to pack a carry-on bag with:

- All medicines including over-the-counter products needed for the entire trip. It is a good idea to bring extra. Keep all medicines in their original containers.
- List of current medicines including brand/generic name and dose. Drug formulations vary from country to country.
- Copy of your electrocardiogram (EKG).
- Name and contact information for your doctors and family members.
- Doctor's letter describing your medical history and any special concerns such as the use of Coumadin™, pacemaker or implanted defibrillator.
- Your personal and emergency medical identification.

Notes

MONDAY

Minutes of exercise _____
Weight _____
Blood pressure _____

TUESDAY

Minutes of exercise _____
Weight _____
Blood pressure _____

WEDNESDAY

Minutes of exercise _____
Weight _____
Blood pressure _____

THURSDAY

Minutes of exercise _____
Weight _____
Blood pressure _____

FRIDAY

Minutes of exercise _____
Weight _____
Blood pressure _____

SATURDAY

Minutes of exercise _____
Weight _____
Blood pressure _____

SUNDAY

Minutes of exercise _____
Weight _____
Blood pressure _____

Things to do for next week:

Check next week's supply of:
- ○ blood pressure medication
- ○ cholesterol medication
- ○ aspirin
- ○ vitamins
- ○ diabetes medication
- ○ lancets
- ○ glucose test strips

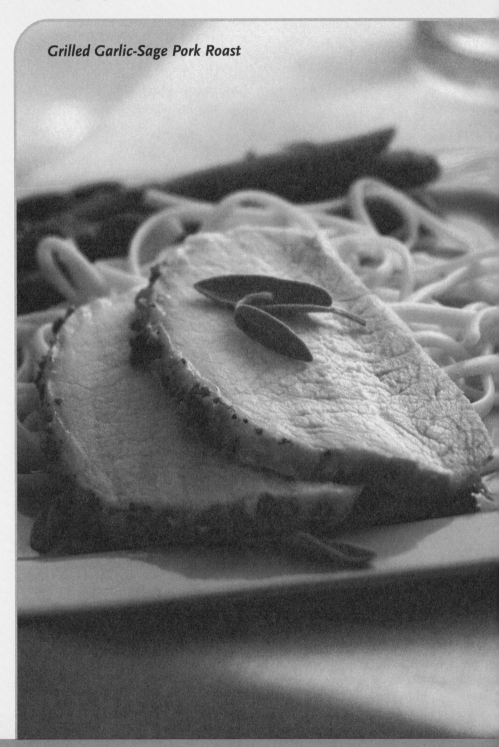

Grilled Garlic-Sage Pork Roast

Grilled Garlic-Sage Pork Roast

PREP: 15 min GRILL: 40 min STAND: 10 min
6 servings

Ingredients
8 cloves garlic, finely chopped
3 tablespoons chopped fresh sage leaves
1/2 teaspoon salt
1/4 teaspoon pepper
2 tablespoons olive or canola oil
1 1/2-pound boneless center-cut pork loin roast

1   Brush grill rack with canola or soybean oil. Heat coals or gas
    grill for direct heat. Mix garlic, sage, salt, pepper and oil in
    small bowl; rub over pork.

2   Cover and grill pork 4 to 5 inches from
    medium heat 35 to 40 minutes, turning
    occasionally, until meat thermometer
    inserted into center of pork reads 155°.
    Remove from heat; cover with aluminum
    foil and let stand 10 minutes until
    thermometer reads 160°. Cut pork across
    grain into thin slices.

To bake in oven, *heat oven to 400°;*
place pork in ungreased rectangular pan,
13 x 9 x 2 inches. Bake 50 to 60 minutes
or until meat thermometer inserted into
center of pork reads 155°. Remove from
oven; cover with aluminum foil and let
stand 10 minutes until thermometer
reads 160°.

1 Serving:

Calories 220
(Calories from Fat 115)
Fat 13g
Saturated Fat 4g
(15% of Calories from
 Saturated Fat)
Trans Fat 0g
Cholesterol 75mg
Omega-3 0g
Sodium 180mg

Exchanges:
4 Lean Meat

3 Carbohydrate Choices

High Blood Pressure

What is blood pressure? Blood pressure can be defined by this formula: Blood Pressure = Blood flowing through the artery (cardiac output) X the stiffness of the artery wall (vascular resistance).

When either excess blood volume or vascular resistance is present, your heart must work harder to pump blood through the arteries. This leads to high blood pressure (hypertension). Because there are no symptoms, many people do not even realize they have high blood pressure. It has sometimes been called the "silent killer."

Be sure to read food labels to identify foods high in salt. Try to avoid "side items" with more than 250 mg of sodium and "entrees" with more than 500 mg of sodium.

Try to limit fast foods or processed foods that are high in sodium. Check the labels of packaged foods for their sodium content.

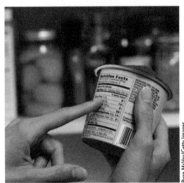

Ryan McVay/Getty Images

Notes

MONDAY

Minutes of exercise _____
Weight _____
Blood pressure _____

TUESDAY

Minutes of exercise _____
Weight _____
Blood pressure _____

WEDNESDAY

Minutes of exercise _____
Weight _____
Blood pressure _____

THURSDAY

Minutes of exercise _____
Weight _____
Blood pressure _____

FRIDAY

Minutes of exercise _____
Weight _____
Blood pressure _____

SATURDAY

Minutes of exercise _____
Weight _____
Blood pressure _____

SUNDAY

Minutes of exercise _____
Weight _____
Blood pressure _____

Things to do for next week:

Check next week's supply of:
- ○ blood pressure medication
- ○ cholesterol medication
- ○ aspirin
- ○ vitamins
- ○ diabetes medication
- ○ lancets
- ○ glucose test strips

Lemon- and Wine-Baked Halibut

PREP: 5 min BAKE: 25 min
4 servings

Ingredients
4 halibut, swordfish or tuna fillets, about 1 inch thick (about 1 1/2 pounds)
1/4 teaspoon salt
4 sprigs dill weed
4 slices lemon
4 black peppercorns
1/4 cup dry white wine or chicken broth

1 Heat oven to 450°. Place fish in ungreased rectangular baking dish, 11 x 7 x 1 1/2 inches. Sprinkle with salt. Place dill weed sprig and lemon slice on each. Top with peppercorns. Pour wine over fish.

2 Bake uncovered 20 to 25 minutes or until fish flakes easily with fork.

1 Serving:

Calories 145
(Calories from Fat 20)
Fat 2g
Saturated Fat 0g
(2% of Calories from Saturated Fat)
Trans Fat 0g
Cholesterol 90mg
Omega-3 1g
Sodium 290mg

Exchanges:
2 Starch, 1 Fat

0 Carbohydrate Choices

Summer Harvest Chicken-Potato Salad

PREP: 15 min
4 servings

Ingredients
4 medium red potatoes (1 pound), cut into 3/4-inch cubes
1/2 pound fresh green beans, trimmed, cut into 1-inch pieces (about 2 cups)
1/2 cup fat-free plain yogurt
1/3 cup fat-free ranch dressing
1 tablespoon prepared horseradish
1/4 teaspoon salt
Dash of pepper
2 cups cut-up cooked chicken breast
2/3 cup thinly sliced celery
Torn salad greens, if desired

1 Heat 6 cups lightly salted water to boiling in 2-quart saucepan. Add potatoes; return to boiling. Reduce heat; simmer 5 minutes. Add green beans; cook uncovered 8 to 12 minutes longer or until potatoes and beans are crisp-tender.

2 Meanwhile, mix yogurt, dressing, horseradish, salt and pepper in small bowl; set aside.

3 Drain potatoes and green beans; rinse with cold water to cool. Mix potatoes, green beans, chicken and celery in large serving bowl. Pour yogurt mixture over salad; toss gently to coat. Line plates with greens; spoon salad onto greens.

1 Serving:

Calories 145
(Calories from Fat 45)
Fat 5g
Saturated Fat 2g
(11% of Calories from Saturated Fat)
Trans Fat 0g
Cholesterol 0mg
Omega-3 0g
Sodium 40mg

Exchanges:
2 Starch, 2 Very Lean Meat, 2 Vegetable

2.5 Carbohydrate Choices

Attitude

Heart disease is serious, but with a positive attitude and discipline, you can make the necessary changes that can lead to an active, healthy life.

Start by being honest with yourself. You have to want to control your blood pressure, weight, and cholesterol levels — which all take discipline. Start by listening to your doctor and asking questions if you do not understand your treatment options. If you need to take medications, be sure that you take them on a regularly scheduled basis.

To control your weight, you may need to meet with a registered dietitian for advice on modifying your current diet. A major factor for most people with heart disease is learning to control portion size at meal time.

Most importantly, you doctor may recommend an exercise program. Be patient with your progress — don't expect to achieve results in the first week or two. Stick with your program, try to exercise for a minimum of 10 minutes every day, and gradually increase the amount of time you exercise.

While you may never be able to completely reverse your condition, by controlling your weight, blood pressure, and cholesterol, you will be better able to put heart disease in its proper perspective — allowing yourself to be a person first, and a person with heart disease second.

Courage is being scared to death and saddling up anyway.
—John Wayne

Notes

MONDAY

Minutes of exercise _____
Weight _____
Blood pressure _____

TUESDAY

Minutes of exercise _____
Weight _____
Blood pressure _____

WEDNESDAY

Minutes of exercise _____
Weight _____
Blood pressure _____

THURSDAY

Minutes of exercise _____
Weight _____
Blood pressure _____

FRIDAY

Minutes of exercise _____
Weight _____
Blood pressure _____

SATURDAY

Minutes of exercise _____
Weight _____
Blood pressure _____

SUNDAY

Minutes of exercise _____
Weight _____
Blood pressure _____

Things to do for next week:

Check next week's supply of:
- ○ blood pressure medication
- ○ cholesterol medication
- ○ aspirin
- ○ vitamins
- ○ diabetes medication
- ○ lancets
- ○ glucose test strips

Roasted Sesame and Honey Snack Mix

PREP: 15 min BAKE: 40 min COOL: 10 min
20 servings (1/2 cup each)

Ingredients
3 cups Wheat Chex® cereal
3 cups checkerboard-shaped pretzels
2 cups popped light microwave popcorn
1 cup sesame sticks
1 cup mixed nuts
1/4 cup honey
3 tablespoons canola or soybean oil
2 tablespoons sesame seed, toasted, if desired*

*To quickly toast sesame seed, cook in a small nonstick skillet over medium heat 1 to 3 minutes, stirring frequently, until light golden brown.

1 Heat oven to 275°. Mix cereal, pretzels, popcorn, sesame sticks and nuts in ungreased jelly roll pan, 15 1/2 x 10 1/2 x 1 inch.

2 Mix remaining ingredients in small bowl. Pour over cereal mixture, stirring until evenly coated.

3 Bake 45 minutes, stirring occasionally. Spread on waxed paper; cool about 30 minutes. Store in tightly covered container up to 1 week.

1/2 Cup:

Calories 165
(Calories from Fat 35)
Fat 4g
Saturated Fat 0g
(3% of Calories from
Saturated Fat)
Trans Fat 0g
Cholesterol 0mg
Omega-3 0g
Sodium 440mg

Exchanges:
1 Starch, 1 Other
Carbohydrates, 1/2 Fat

2.5 Carbohydrate Choices

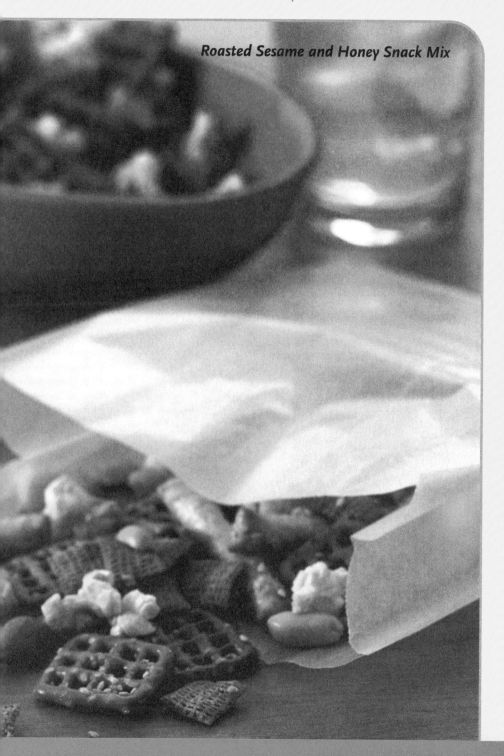

Roasted Sesame and Honey Snack Mix

Smoking

Smoking and heart disease do not mix. Smoking introduces carbon monoxide into the body. Carbon monoxide robs oxygen from the heart, muscles, and body.

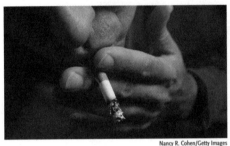

People who smoke increase their risk of developing heart disease and many other serious illnesses.

Nancy R. Cohen/Getty Images

Because it reduces the "good" HDL-cholesterol and makes the blood clot more easily, smoking increases the risk of heart attack or stroke. It is also a risk factor for blockages of the arteries to the brain, kidneys, and legs.

There is no such thing in anyone's life as an unimportant day.
—Alexander Wolcott

Notes

MONDAY

Minutes of exercise _____
Weight _____
Blood pressure _____

TUESDAY

Minutes of exercise _____
Weight _____
Blood pressure _____

WEDNESDAY

Minutes of exercise _____
Weight _____
Blood pressure _____

THURSDAY

Minutes of exercise _____
Weight _____
Blood pressure _____

FRIDAY

Minutes of exercise _____
Weight _____
Blood pressure _____

SATURDAY

Minutes of exercise _____
Weight _____
Blood pressure _____

SUNDAY

Minutes of exercise _____
Weight _____
Blood pressure _____

Things to do for next week:

Check next week's supply of:
- ○ blood pressure medication
- ○ cholesterol medication
- ○ aspirin
- ○ vitamins
- ○ diabetes medication
- ○ lancets
- ○ glucose test strips

Springtime Pasta and Sausage

PREP: 10 min COOK: 15 min
6 servings

Ingredients

1/2 teaspoon fennel seed
5 roma (plum) tomatoes, chopped
1/3 cup chopped fresh parsley
4 medium green onions, cut into 1-inch pieces
2 cups sliced fresh mushrooms (about 5 ounces)
8 ounces uncooked regular or whole-wheat spaghetti
12 ounces Italian turkey sausage links, thinly sliced
1 package (9 ounces) frozen sugar snap peas in a pouch, thawed

2 cloves garlic, minced
1/3 cup chicken broth

1 Cook spaghetti as directed on package in 4-quart Dutch oven or saucepan; drain and return to Dutch oven.

2 Meanwhile, cook sausage, fennel and garlic in 10-inch nonstick skillet over medium heat, stirring frequently, until sausage is no longer pink in center; drain. Remove sausage from skillet.

3 Place sugar snap peas, mushrooms and broth in skillet. Heat to boiling; reduce heat to medium-low. Simmer uncovered 3 to 4 minutes, stirring frequently. Stir in tomatoes and green onions; cook over medium heat, stirring frequently, about 2 minutes. Add sausage and parsley; cook 1 minute longer or until hot.

4 Add sausage mixture to spaghetti in Dutch oven; toss gently to mix.

1 Serving:

Calories 145
(Calories from Fat 20)
Fat 2g
Saturated Fat 0g
(2% of Calories from Saturated Fat)
Trans Fat 0g
Cholesterol 90mg
Omega-3 1g
Sodium 290mg

Exchanges:
2 Starch, 1 Fat

2.5 Carbohydrate Choices

Gorgonzola Linguine with Toasted Walnuts

PREP: 10 min   COOK: 15 min
6 servings

Ingredients
4 ounces uncooked linguine
1 tablespoon butter
1 clove garlic, crushed
1 tablespoon all-purpose flour
1 cup evaporated skimmed milk
1/4 cup dry white wine or chicken broth
1/4 teaspoon salt
1/2 cup crumbled Gorgonzola cheese (2 ounces)
3 tablespoons walnuts, toasted and finely chopped*

*To toast nuts, bake uncovered in ungreased shallow pan in 350° oven about
10 minutes, stirring occasionally, until golden brown. Or cook in ungreased
heavy skillet over medium-low heat 5 to 7 minutes, stirring frequently until
browning begins, then stirring constantly until golden brown.

1   Cook and drain linguine as directed on
    package.

2   Meanwhile, melt butter in 2-quart saucepan
    over medium heat. Cook garlic in butter,
    stirring occasionally, until garlic is golden
    brown. Stir in flour until smooth and
    bubbly. Stir in milk, wine and salt. Cook,
    stirring constantly, until mixture begins to
    thicken.

3   Reduce heat to medium-low. Stir cheese
    into sauce; cook, stirring frequently, until
    cheese is melted. Toss linguine and sauce
    in large bowl. Sprinkle with walnuts.

1 Serving:

Calories 185
(Calories from Fat 65)
Fat 7g
Saturated Fat 3g
(16% of Calories from
Saturated Fat)
Trans Fat 0g
Cholesterol 15mg
Omega-3 0g
Sodium 200mg

Exchanges:
1 1/2 Starch, 1/2
High-Fat Meat, 1/2 Fat

1.5 Carbohydrate Choices

Heart Health

According to the American Heart Association, people who have heart disease are six times more likely to have another cardiovascular event (heart attack, stroke, angioplasty or bypass surgery) than people without heart disease are to have their first event. To reduce your risk of having a second event, you should:

- Stop smoking
- Exercise regularly
- Follow a healthy diet
- Maintain proper weight

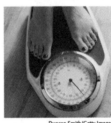

Watch your weight.

Duncan Smith/Getty Images

Schedule regular medical checkups and record your cholesterol, blood pressure readings, weight, and blood sugar (if necessary). If you have abnormal values for any of these measures, medication might help. Follow your doctor's instructions and be sure to ask your doctor for clarification if you have any questions.

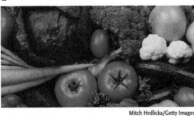

Eat plenty of fresh fruits and vegetables daily.

Mitch Hrdlicka/Getty Images

Exercise regularly.

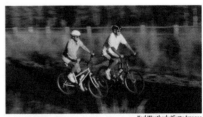

Karl Weatherly/Getty Images

If you risk nothing, then you risk everything.
—Geena Davis

Notes

MONDAY

Minutes of exercise _____
Weight _____
Blood pressure _____

TUESDAY

Minutes of exercise _____
Weight _____
Blood pressure _____

WEDNESDAY

Minutes of exercise _____
Weight _____
Blood pressure _____

THURSDAY

Minutes of exercise _____
Weight _____
Blood pressure _____

FRIDAY

Minutes of exercise _____
Weight _____
Blood pressure _____

SATURDAY

Minutes of exercise _____
Weight _____
Blood pressure _____

SUNDAY

Minutes of exercise _____
Weight _____
Blood pressure _____

Things to do for next week:

Check next week's supply of:
○ blood pressure medication
○ cholesterol medication
○ aspirin
○ vitamins
○ diabetes medication
○ lancets
○ glucose test strips

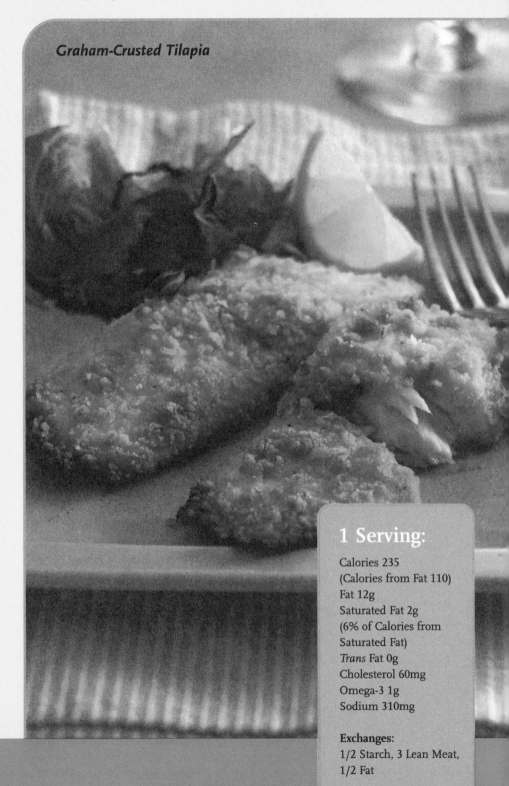

Graham-Crusted Tilapia

1 Serving:

Calories 235
(Calories from Fat 110)
Fat 12g
Saturated Fat 2g
(6% of Calories from
Saturated Fat)
Trans Fat 0g
Cholesterol 60mg
Omega-3 1g
Sodium 310mg

Exchanges:
1/2 Starch, 3 Lean Meat,
1/2 Fat

Graham-Crusted Tilapia

PREP: 15 min   BAKE: 10 min
4 servings

Ingredients
1 pound tilapia, cod, haddock or other medium-firm fish fillets, about
   3/4 inch thick
1/2 cup graham cracker crumbs (about 8 squares)
1 teaspoon grated lemon peel
1/4 teaspoon salt
1/8 teaspoon pepper
1/4 cup milk
2 tablespoons canola or soybean oil
2 tablespoons chopped toasted pecans*

*To toast nuts, bake uncovered in ungreased shallow pan in 350° oven about
10 minutes, stirring occasionally, until golden brown. Or cook in ungreased
heavy skillet over medium-low heat 5 to 7 minutes, stirring frequently until
browning begins, then stirring constantly until golden brown.

1 Move oven rack to position slightly above middle of oven.
   Heat oven to 500°.

2 Cut fish fillets crosswise into 2-inch-wide pieces. Mix cracker
   crumbs, lemon peel, salt and pepper in shallow dish. Place
   milk in another shallow dish.

3 Dip fish into milk, then coat with cracker mixture; place in
   ungreased rectangular pan, 13 x 9 x 2 inches. Drizzle oil over
   fish; sprinkle with pecans.

4 Bake uncovered about 10 minutes or until fish flakes easily
   with fork.

3 Carbohydrate Choices

Tips for Eating Out

Eating at a restaurant can be an enjoyable yet overwhelming experience, especially if you are trying to make healthy selections. Here are some tips for ordering pleasurable and healthy food at a restaurant.

- Choose a restaurant with a diverse menu. There are often more healthy selections from which you can choose.
- Split an entrée with your companion or take half of the entrée home.
- Choose foods that have been baked, broiled, grilled, steamed, or roasted.
- Ask for condiments on the side.
- If you are tempted to fill up on bread and butter, ask the server to remove the basket from the table.
- Choose broth-based soups or a salad as an appetizer. They will make you feel full without providing an excess of calories.
- Make special requests of the chef. Most chefs are willing to accommodate your needs.

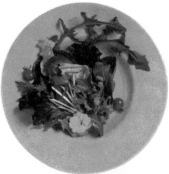

Select a salad as a healthy appetizer.

C Squared Studios/Getty Images

Whether you think you can or think you can't — you are right.
—Henry Ford

Notes

MONDAY

Minutes of exercise _____
Weight _____
Blood pressure _____

TUESDAY

Minutes of exercise _____
Weight _____
Blood pressure _____

WEDNESDAY

Minutes of exercise _____
Weight _____
Blood pressure _____

THURSDAY

Minutes of exercise _____
Weight _____
Blood pressure _____

FRIDAY

Minutes of exercise _____
Weight _____
Blood pressure _____

SATURDAY

Minutes of exercise _____
Weight _____
Blood pressure _____

SUNDAY

Minutes of exercise _____
Weight _____
Blood pressure _____

Things to do for next week:

Check next week's supply of:
○ blood pressure medication
○ cholesterol medication
○ aspirin
○ vitamins
○ diabetes medication
○ lancets
○ glucose test strips

Tropical Fruit, Rice and Tuna Salad

PREP: 15 min COOK: 10 min COOL: 15 min CHILL: 3 hrs
4 servings

Ingredients
1 cup water
3/4 cup uncooked instant brown rice
1/2 cup vanilla low-fat yogurt
1 can (8 ounces) pineapple tidbits in juice, drained and 1 teaspoon
    juice reserved
2 kiwifruit, peeled and sliced
1 medium mango, peeled, seeded and chopped (about 1 cup)
1 can (6 ounces) white tuna in water, drained and flaked
1 tablespoon coconut, toasted*

*To toast coconut, bake uncovered in ungreased shallow pan in 350° oven
5 to 7 minutes, stirring occasionally, until golden brown. Or cook in
ungreased heavy skillet over medium-low heat 6 to 14 minutes, stirring
frequently until browning begins, then stirring constantly until golden brown.

1 Heat water to boiling in 1-quart saucepan. Stir in rice; reduce
   heat to low. Cover and simmer 10 minutes. Uncover; cool
   15 minutes. Refrigerate at least 1 hour or until cold.

2 Mix rice, yogurt and reserved
   pineapple juice in medium bowl.
   Cover and refrigerate 1 to 2 hours
   to blend flavors.

3 Cut kiwifruit slices into fourths.
   Gently stir kiwifruit, pineapple,
   mango and tuna into rice mixture.
   Sprinkle with coconut.

1 Serving:

Calories 260
(Calories from Fat 20)
Fat 2g
Saturated Fat 1g
(3% of Calories from
Saturated Fat)
Trans Fat 0g
Cholesterol 15mg
Omega-3 0g
Sodium 170mg

Exchanges: 2 Starch,
1 Fruit, 1 1/2 Very
Lean Meat

3 Carbohydrate Choices

Chocolate-Filled Cake Roll

PREP: 25 min BAKE: 13 min COOL: 45 min CHILL: 2 hrs
12 servings

Ingredients

1/4 cup powdered sugar	3 eggs
1 cup granulated sugar	1/3 cup water
1 cup all-purpose flour	1 teaspoon baking powder
1 cup fat-free (skim) milk	1/4 teaspoon salt
2 tablespoons miniature chocolate chips	1 teaspoon vanilla

1 cup frozen (thawed) fat-free whipped topping
1 package (4-serving size) chocolate fat-free sugar-free instant pudding and
  pie filling mix

1 Heat oven to 375°. Line jelly roll pan, 15 1/2 x 10 1/2 x 1 inch, with waxed paper. Grease waxed paper with shortening; lightly flour. Sprinkle powdered sugar evenly over clean dish towel in a rectangle the same size as the pan.

2 Beat eggs with balloon whisk or electric mixer with regular beaters on medium speed about 3 minutes or until thick and lemon colored. Beat in granulated sugar, water and vanilla. Beat in flour, baking powder and salt on low speed, mixing just until combined. Pour into pan. Sprinkle with chocolate chips.

3 Bake 11 to 13 minutes or until toothpick inserted in center comes out clean and top is just beginning to brown. Run knife around edges of pan to loosen cake. Immediately turn pan upside down onto sugared towel; remove pan and carefully peel off waxed paper. Place clean sheet of waxed paper over top of hot cake; gently roll up cake in towel starting with one long side. Cool at least 45 minutes.

4 Stir pudding mix (dry) and milk in medium bowl with wire whisk or fork 1 to 2 minutes or until thickened. Fold in whipped topping. Unroll cake and spread pudding mixture to within 1/2 inch of edges. Reroll cake. Wrap in plastic wrap; refrigerate at least 2 hours for filling to set. Store in refrigerator.

2 Carbohydrate Choices

Exercise

Exercise is a very important tool for controlling heart disease.

Because everyone is different, you should obtain approval from your doctor before you begin a "vigorous" exercise routine. Almost everyone can start with a simple exercise program and build up gradually.

Also, for a person with both heart disease and type 1 diabetes, food and insulin regimens may have to be changed to provide enough energy for exercise. Your diabetes educator or dietitian can help you with any changes.

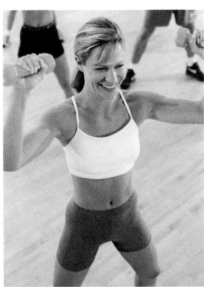

Ryan McVay/Getty Images

Talk to your doctor about exercise. Most likely he or she will recommend that you start with a simple routine and build up gradually.

The men who try to do something and fail are infinitely better than those who try to do nothing and succeed.
                                                                    —Lloyd Jones

Notes

MONDAY

Minutes of exercise _____
Weight _____
Blood pressure _____

TUESDAY

Minutes of exercise _____
Weight _____
Blood pressure _____

WEDNESDAY

Minutes of exercise _____
Weight _____
Blood pressure _____

THURSDAY

Minutes of exercise _____
Weight _____
Blood pressure _____

FRIDAY

Minutes of exercise _____
Weight _____
Blood pressure _____

SATURDAY

Minutes of exercise _____
Weight _____
Blood pressure _____

SUNDAY

Minutes of exercise _____
Weight _____
Blood pressure _____

Things to do for next week:

Check next week's supply of:
- ○ blood pressure medication
- ○ cholesterol medication
- ○ aspirin
- ○ vitamins
- ○ diabetes medication
- ○ lancets
- ○ glucose test strips

Mixed-Berry Coffee Cake

PREP: 15 min BAKE: 33 min COOL: 10 min
8 servings

Ingredients
1/3 cup packed brown sugar
1/2 cup buttermilk
2 tablespoons canola or soybean oil
1 teaspoon vanilla
1 egg
1 cup whole wheat flour
1/2 teaspoon baking soda
1/2 teaspoon ground cinnamon
1/8 teaspoon salt
1 cup mixed berries, such as blueberries, raspberries and blackberries
1/4 cup low-fat granola, slightly crushed

1 Heat oven to 350°. Spray round pan, 8 x 1 1/2 or
   9 x 1 1/2 inches, with cooking spray.

2 Mix brown sugar, buttermilk, oil, vanilla and egg in large bowl
   until smooth. Stir in flour, baking soda, cinnamon and salt
   just until moistened. Gently fold in half of the berries. Spoon
   into pan. Sprinkle with remaining berries and the granola.

3 Bake 28 to 33 minutes or until
   golden brown and top springs
   back when touched in center.
   Cool in pan on wire rack
   10 minutes. Serve warm.

1 Serving:

Calories 150
(Calories from Fat 45)
Fat 5g
Saturated Fat 1g
(4% of Calories from
Saturated Fat)
Trans Fat 0g
Cholesterol 25mg
Omega-3 0g
Sodium 150mg

Exchanges:
1 Starch, 1/2 Fruit, 1 Fat

2.5 Carbohydrate Choices

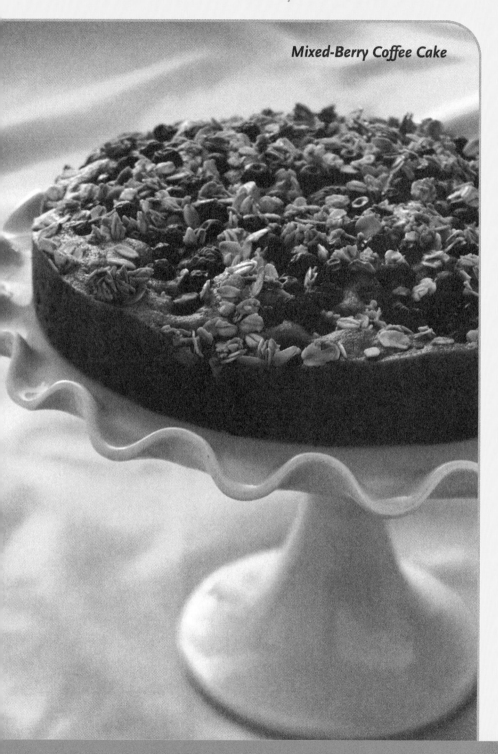

Mixed-Berry Coffee Cake

Emergency Medical ID

Carrying medical identification could save your life. You should carry information identifying your medical conditions (i.e., type of heart condition, pacemaker/defibrillator or Coumadin™ use) on a medical alert necklace or bracelet and on a card that can be carried in your pocket or wallet. This helps emergency personnel work quickly to provide proper care.

Be sure your identification is easy to find. Emergency personnel typically look for necklaces and bracelets first. However, watch charms, shoe tags, and ankle bracelets are also options.

We can do anything we want to do if we stick to it long enough.
—Helen Keller

Notes

MONDAY

Minutes of exercise _____
Weight _____
Blood pressure _____

TUESDAY

Minutes of exercise _____
Weight _____
Blood pressure _____

WEDNESDAY

Minutes of exercise _____
Weight _____
Blood pressure _____

THURSDAY

Minutes of exercise _____
Weight _____
Blood pressure _____

FRIDAY

Minutes of exercise _____
Weight _____
Blood pressure _____

SATURDAY

Minutes of exercise _____
Weight _____
Blood pressure _____

SUNDAY

Minutes of exercise _____
Weight _____
Blood pressure _____

Things to do for next week:

Check next week's supply of:
- ○ blood pressure medication
- ○ cholesterol medication
- ○ aspirin
- ○ vitamins
- ○ diabetes medication
- ○ lancets
- ○ glucose test strips

Buckwheat-Orange Waffles

PREP: 10 min BAKE: 5 min per waffle
6 servings

Ingredients
1 egg
1/2 cup fat-free (skim) milk
1/2 cup plain nonfat yogurt
2 teaspoons grated orange peel
1 cup orange juice (about 2 medium oranges)
1 cup buckwheat flour
3/4 cup all-purpose flour
2 teaspoons baking powder
1 teaspoon baking soda
1/4 teaspoon ground cloves

1   Spray nonstick waffle iron with cooking spray; heat waffle iron. Place all ingredients in blender or food processor. Cover and blend until smooth.

2   For each waffle, pour 1/2 cup batter onto center of hot waffle iron; close lid. Bake 4 to 5 minutes or until steaming stops. Carefully remove waffle.

1 Serving:

Calories 180
(Calories from Fat 20)
Fat 2g
Saturated Fat 0g
(3% of Calories from
Saturated Fat)
Trans Fat 0g
Cholesterol 35mg
Omega-3 0g
Sodium 410mg

Exchanges:
2 Starch, 1/2 Fat

2 Carbohydrate Choices

Campfire Popcorn Snack

PREP: 5 min   BAKE: 10 min 12 servings
About 20 servings (1/2 cup each)

Ingredients
6 cups popped light butter-flavor microwave popcorn
4 cups Wheat, Corn or Rice Chex® cereal
1 jar (7 ounces) marshmallow creme

1   Heat oven to 350°. Spray cookie sheet with cooking spray.
    Mix popcorn and cereal in large bowl; set aside.

2   Microwave marshmallow creme in medium
    microwavable bowl uncovered on High
    1 minute; stir. Microwave about 1 minute
    longer or until melted; stir. Pour over
    popcorn mixture, stirring until evenly
    coated. Spread mixture on cookie sheet.

3   Bake 5 minutes; stir. Bake about 5 minutes
    longer or until coating is light golden
    brown. Spread on waxed paper or
    aluminum foil to cool. Store in tightly
    covered container up to 2 weeks.

1/2 Cup:

Calories 65
(Calories from Fat 0)
Fat 0g
Saturated Fat 0g
(3% of Calories from
Saturated Fat)
Trans Fat 0g
Cholesterol 0mg
Omega-3 0g
Sodium 90mg

Exchanges:
1 Other Carbohydrates

1 Carbohydrate Choice

Vascular Inflammation and C-Reactive Protein

Vascular inflammation is another risk factor for cardiovascular disease. Smoking, high cholesterol, high blood pressure and diabetes can all result in inflammation, which then causes plaque to grow in the artery walls. If the plaque ruptures, blood clots can form, leading to increased risk for heart attack or chest pain.

Your doctor may order a simple blood test to check your C-reactive protein (CRP) levels, which can reflect the degree of vascular inflammation.

You can reduce your CRP levels by losing weight, closely controlling diabetes, exercising regularly and quitting smoking. Certain medications – such as aspirin, statins, ACE-inhibitors and others – are also effective in lowering CRP levels.

Only the mediocre are always at their best.
—Jean Giraudoux

Notes

MONDAY

Minutes of exercise _____
Weight _____
Blood pressure _____

TUESDAY

Minutes of exercise _____
Weight _____
Blood pressure _____

WEDNESDAY

Minutes of exercise _____
Weight _____
Blood pressure _____

THURSDAY

Minutes of exercise _____
Weight _____
Blood pressure _____

FRIDAY

Minutes of exercise _____
Weight _____
Blood pressure _____

SATURDAY

Minutes of exercise _____
Weight _____
Blood pressure _____

SUNDAY

Minutes of exercise _____
Weight _____
Blood pressure _____

Things to do for next week:

Check next week's supply of:
- ○ vitamins
- ○ blood pressure medication
- ○ diabetes medication
- ○ cholesterol medication
- ○ lancets
- ○ aspirin
- ○ glucose test strips

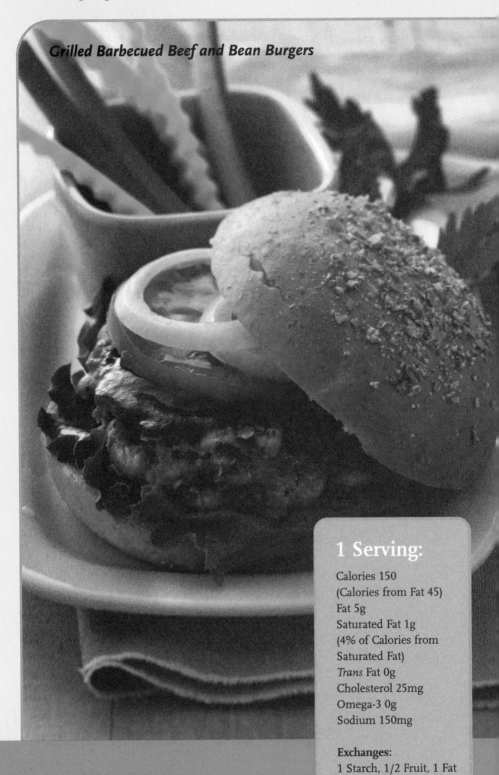

Grilled Barbecued Beef and Bean Burgers

1 Serving:

Calories 150
(Calories from Fat 45)
Fat 5g
Saturated Fat 1g
(4% of Calories from
Saturated Fat)
Trans Fat 0g
Cholesterol 25mg
Omega-3 0g
Sodium 150mg

Exchanges:
1 Starch, 1/2 Fruit, 1 Fat

Grilled Barbecued Beef and Bean Burgers

PREP: 10 min   GRILL: 13 min
5 servings

Ingredients
1/2 pound extra-lean ground beef
1 can (15 to 16 ounces) great northern beans, rinsed and drained
1/4 cup finely crushed saltine crackers (about 7 squares)
2 tablespoons barbecue sauce
1/4 teaspoon pepper
1 egg
5 teaspoons barbecue sauce
5 whole-grain hamburger buns, split
Leaf lettuce, sliced tomatoes and sliced onions, if desired

1   Brush grill rack with canola or soybean oil. Heat coals or gas grill for direct heat.

2   Mix beef, beans, cracker crumbs, 2 tablespoons barbecue sauce, the pepper and egg in large bowl. Shape mixture into 5 patties, about 1/2 inch thick.

3   Cover and grill patties 4 to 6 inches from medium heat 5 minutes. Turn patties; spread each patty with 1 teaspoon barbecue sauce. Grill until meat thermometer inserted in center of patties reads 160°, about 6 to 8 minutes longer.

4   Fill buns with lettuce, patties, tomatoes and onions.

3 Carbohydrate Choices

Healthy Holiday Eating

The holiday season is a very busy and enjoyable time of year. Many holiday activities involve eating. Consequently, controlling your blood sugar during this time can be difficult. Here are some tips to help you enjoy your holiday season while managing your diabetes:

- Eat before you go out to prevent overeating high-fat or high-carbohydrate foods at the event.
- Enjoy small portions of your favorite foods.
- Savor the foods that you do eat by eating slowly.
- Try to eat at your normal meal times.
- Participate in holiday activities that don't revolve around eating. For example, when you are visiting family and relatives, try to get a group to go for a walk.
- Stick to your exercise plan.

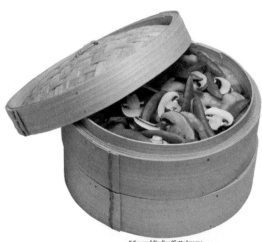

Offer to bring a healthy covered dish, such as vegetables, to the event.

C Squared Studios/Getty Images

Never eat more than you can lift.
—Miss Piggy

Notes

MONDAY

Minutes of exercise _____
Weight _____
Blood pressure _____

TUESDAY

Minutes of exercise _____
Weight _____
Blood pressure _____

WEDNESDAY

Minutes of exercise _____
Weight _____
Blood pressure _____

THURSDAY

Minutes of exercise _____
Weight _____
Blood pressure _____

FRIDAY

Minutes of exercise _____
Weight _____
Blood pressure _____

SATURDAY

Minutes of exercise _____
Weight _____
Blood pressure _____

SUNDAY

Minutes of exercise _____
Weight _____
Blood pressure _____

Things to do for next week:

Check next week's supply of:
- ○ blood pressure medication
- ○ cholesterol medication
- ○ aspirin
- ○ vitamins
- ○ diabetes medication
- ○ lancets
- ○ glucose test strips

Garlic- and Herb-Broiled Rainbow Trout

PREP: 10 min   BROIL: 4 min
4 servings

Ingredients
4 rainbow trout or other medium-firm fish fillets, 1/4 to 1/2 inch thick (about
   1 pound)
2 tablespoons lime or lemon juice
2/3 cup soft bread crumbs (about 1 slice bread)
1 teaspoon Italian seasoning
2 teaspoons canola or soybean oil
1/2 teaspoon garlic powder
1/4 teaspoon pepper

1   Set oven control to broil. Spray broiler pan rack with cooking
    spray. Place fish on rack in broiler pan. Brush with lime juice.
    Broil with tops about 4 inches from heat 3 minutes.

2   While fish is broiling, mix remaining ingredients.

3   Spoon bread crumb mixture on top of fish. Broil about
    1 minute longer or until fish flakes
    easily with fork.

1 Serving:

Calories 175
(Calories from Fat 70)
Fat 8g
Saturated Fat 2g
(9% of Calories from
Saturated Fat)
Trans Fat 0g
Cholesterol 65mg
Omega-3 2g
Sodium 95mg

Exchanges:
3 Lean Meat

0 Carbohydrate Choices

Border Chicken and Bean Soup

PREP: 10 min COOK: 20 min
6 servings

Ingredients
3/4 pound boneless skinless chicken thighs or breast halves
3 cups fat-free reduced-sodium chicken broth
1 can (15 to 16 ounces) navy beans, rinsed and drained
1 can (14 1/2 ounces) no-salt-added diced tomatoes, undrained
1 envelope (1 1/4 ounces) taco seasoning mix
1 1/2 teaspoons sugar

1   Cut chicken into 1/2-inch pieces. Spray 4-quart Dutch oven
    with cooking spray; heat over medium-high heat. Cook
    chicken in Dutch oven about 3 minutes, stirring frequently,
    until brown.

2   Stir in remaining ingredients. Heat to
    boiling; reduce heat to low. Simmer
    uncovered about 15 minutes or until
    chicken is no longer pink in center.

1/2 Cup:

Calories 225
(Calories from Fat 55)
Fat 6g
Saturated Fat 2g
(6% of Calories from
Saturated Fat)
Trans Fat 0g
Cholesterol 35mg
Omega-3 0g
Sodium 790mg

Exchanges:
2 Starch, 2 Very
Lean Meat

2 Carbohydrate Choices

Blood Pressure

Hypertension, or high blood pressure, can complicate heart disease. Two readings of a systolic pressure (the "top number") greater than 130 mm Hg and/or a diastolic pressure (the "bottom number") greater than 80 mm Hg could mean you have high blood pressure.

When an artery expands to handle the blood pumping out of the heart, the pressure put on the artery wall is called systolic pressure. The artery then relaxes back to normal, and the pressure that occurs during relaxation is called diastolic pressure.

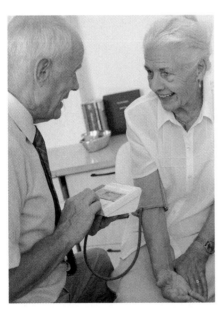

Most likely, your doctor will monitor your blood pressure. In addition, he or she may suggest that you talk to a pharmacist about purchasing a blood pressure monitor for home.

Notes

MONDAY

Minutes of exercise _____
Weight _____
Blood pressure _____

TUESDAY

Minutes of exercise _____
Weight _____
Blood pressure _____

WEDNESDAY

Minutes of exercise _____
Weight _____
Blood pressure _____

THURSDAY

Minutes of exercise _____
Weight _____
Blood pressure _____

FRIDAY

Minutes of exercise _____
Weight _____
Blood pressure _____

SATURDAY

Minutes of exercise _____
Weight _____
Blood pressure _____

SUNDAY

Minutes of exercise _____
Weight _____
Blood pressure _____

Things to do for next week:

Check next week's supply of:
○ blood pressure medication
○ cholesterol medication
○ aspirin
○ vitamins
○ diabetes medication
○ lancets
○ glucose test strips

Gyro Salad

PREP: 20 min   COOK: 5 min
6 servings

Ingredients
Yogurt Dressing (below)
1-pound boneless beef sirloin steak, 1 to 1 1/2 inches thick
1 tablespoon canola or soybean oil
1 1/4 teaspoons Greek seasoning
8 cups torn mixed salad greens
1 medium cucumber, thinly sliced (1 1/2 cups)
1 small red onion, thinly sliced and separated into rings
1 large tomato, chopped (1 cup)

1   Make Yogurt Dressing; set aside.

2   Cut beef across grain into 4 x 1/4-inch strips. Heat oil in 12-inch nonstick skillet over medium-high heat. Add beef to skillet; sprinkle with Greek seasoning. Cook about 5 minutes, stirring frequently, until beef is brown. Drain if necessary.

3   Arrange salad greens on serving platter or individual serving plates. Top with cucumber, onion, tomato and beef. Serve with dressing.

Yogurt Dressing
1/2 cup plain fat-free yogurt
1/2 cup reduced-fat sour cream
1/4 cup fat-free (skim) milk
1 teaspoon Greek seasoning

Mix all ingredients in small bowl with wire whisk until creamy.

2.5 Carbohydrate Choices

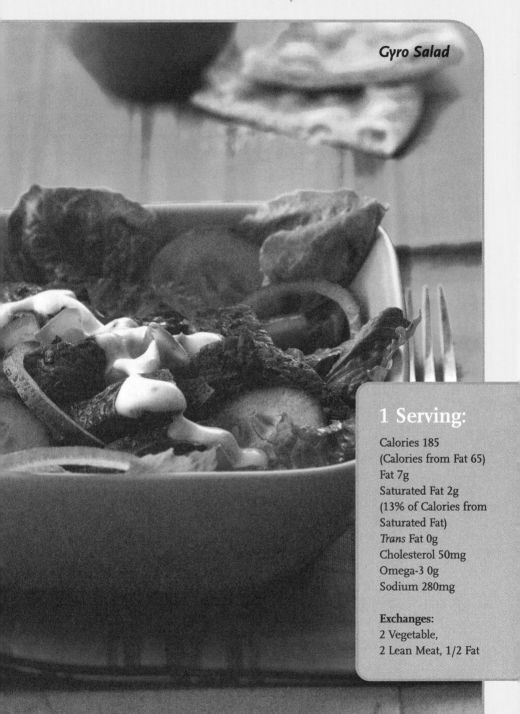

Gyro Salad

1 Serving:

Calories 185
(Calories from Fat 65)
Fat 7g
Saturated Fat 2g
(13% of Calories from
Saturated Fat)
Trans Fat 0g
Cholesterol 50mg
Omega-3 0g
Sodium 280mg

Exchanges:
2 Vegetable,
2 Lean Meat, 1/2 Fat

Cholesterol

If you have diabetes, what should your cholesterol numbers be?

Total cholesterol: less than 200 mg/dL
LDL-cholesterol: less than 70 mg/dL if you have heart disease
less than 100 mg/dL if you do not have heart disease
Triglycerides: less than 150 mg/dL
HDL-cholesterol: more than 40 mg/dL for men
more than 50 mg/dL for women

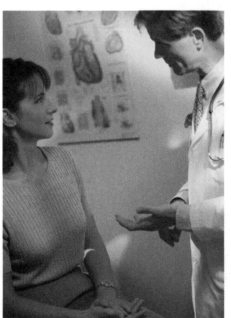

Photodisc Collection/Getty Images

Discuss your most recent cholesterol results with your doctor.

Notes

MONDAY

Minutes of exercise _____
Weight _____
Blood pressure _____

TUESDAY

Minutes of exercise _____
Weight _____
Blood pressure _____

WEDNESDAY

Minutes of exercise _____
Weight _____
Blood pressure _____

THURSDAY

Minutes of exercise _____
Weight _____
Blood pressure _____

FRIDAY

Minutes of exercise _____
Weight _____
Blood pressure _____

SATURDAY

Minutes of exercise _____
Weight _____
Blood pressure _____

SUNDAY

Minutes of exercise _____
Weight _____
Blood pressure _____

Things to do for next week:

Check next week's supply of:

- ○ blood pressure medication
- ○ cholesterol medication
- ○ aspirin
- ○ vitamins
- ○ diabetes medication
- ○ lancets
- ○ glucose test strips

Rush-Hour Tuna Melts

PREP: 10 min BAKE: 10 min
4 servings (2 sandwiches each)

Ingredients
1 can (6 ounces) solid white tuna in water, drained and flaked
3/4 cup chopped celery
2 tablespoons finely chopped onion
1/2 teaspoon grated lemon peel, if desired
1/3 cup fat-free mayonnaise or salad dressing
4 whole wheat English muffins, split and lightly toasted
8 slices tomato
1 cup shredded reduced-fat Cheddar or Monterey Jack cheese (4 ounces)

1   Heat oven to 350°. Mix tuna, celery, onion, lemon peel and
    mayonnaise in medium bowl.

2   Spread about 3 tablespoons tuna mixture on each English
    muffin half. Top each with tomato slice; sprinkle with
    cheese. Place on ungreased cookie sheet.

3   Bake 8 to 10 minutes or until
    cheese is melted and sandwiches
    are thoroughly heated.

1 Serving:

Calories 265
(Calories from Fat 35)
Fat 4g
Saturated Fat 2g
(6% of Calories from
Saturated Fat)
Trans Fat 0g
Cholesterol 20mg
Omega-3 0g
Sodium 895mg

Exchanges:
2 Starch, 2 1/2 Very
Lean Meat, 1/2 Fat

2 Carbohydrate Choices

Five-Spice Tofu Stir-Fry

PREP: 15 min COOK: 25 min STAND: 10 min
4 servings

Ingredients

1 1/4 cups water	1/4 cup water
1 cup uncooked instant brown rice	1/4 cup stir-fry sauce
3/4 teaspoon five-spice powder	1 tablespoon honey
2 tablespoons orange juice	
1 small red onion, cut into thin wedges	
1 package (14 ounces) firm tofu, cut into 3/4-inch cubes	
1 bag (1 pound) frozen baby bean and carrot blend	

1/2 Cup:

Calories 225
(Calories from Fat 55)
Fat 6g
Saturated Fat 2g
(6% of Calories from
Saturated Fat)
Trans Fat 0g
Cholesterol 35mg
Omega-3 0g
Sodium 790mg

Exchanges:
2 Starch,
2 Very Lean Meat

1 Heat 1 1/4 cups water to boiling in 1-quart saucepan. Stir in rice; reduce heat to low. Cover and simmer 10 minutes.

2 Meanwhile, mix stir-fry sauce, orange juice, honey and five-spice powder in medium bowl. Press tofu between paper towels to absorb excess moisture. Stir tofu into sauce mixture; let stand 10 minutes to marinate.

3 Spray 12-inch nonstick skillet with cooking spray; heat over medium heat. Remove tofu from sauce mixture; reserve sauce mixture. Cook tofu in skillet 3 to 4 minutes, stirring occasionally, just until light golden brown. Remove tofu from skillet.

4 Cook onion in skillet 2 minutes, stirring constantly. Add frozen vegetables and 1/4 cup water. Heat to boiling; reduce heat to medium. Cover and cook 6 to 8 minutes, stirring occasionally, until vegetables are crisp-tender.

5 Stir in reserved sauce mixture and tofu. Cook 2 to 3 minutes, stirring occasionally, until mixture is slightly thickened and hot. Serve over rice.

3 Carbohydrate Choices

Stress

When you are under stress, your brain releases signals that affect your heart rate, blood pressure, and other body reactions. If you are under a lot of stress for long periods of time, your heart rate increases while your arteries tighten or narrow. This results in increased blood pressure as more blood is being forced through less space (the narrowed arteries).

Sometimes, medication is needed to improve blood pressure. Reducing stress and adopting a healthy lifestyle can also help. Try meditation, deep breathing, or listening to soothing music. If you smoke, stop. Manage your weight. And remember that exercising regularly can help anything that ails you. Go for a walk, ride a bike, or take a swim.

Try meditation, deep breathing, or going for a walk as a means to reduce stress.

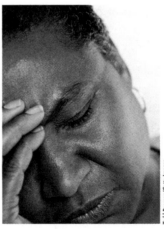

Todd Pearson/Getty Images

If you treat every situation as a life-and-death matter, you'll die a lot of times.
—Dean Smith

Notes

MONDAY

Minutes of exercise _____
Weight _____
Blood pressure _____

TUESDAY

Minutes of exercise _____
Weight _____
Blood pressure _____

WEDNESDAY

Minutes of exercise _____
Weight _____
Blood pressure _____

THURSDAY

Minutes of exercise _____
Weight _____
Blood pressure _____

FRIDAY

Minutes of exercise _____
Weight _____
Blood pressure _____

SATURDAY

Minutes of exercise _____
Weight _____
Blood pressure _____

SUNDAY

Minutes of exercise _____
Weight _____
Blood pressure _____

Things to do for next week:

Check next week's supply of:
- ○ blood pressure medication
- ○ cholesterol medication
- ○ aspirin
- ○ vitamins
- ○ diabetes medication
- ○ lancets
- ○ glucose test strips

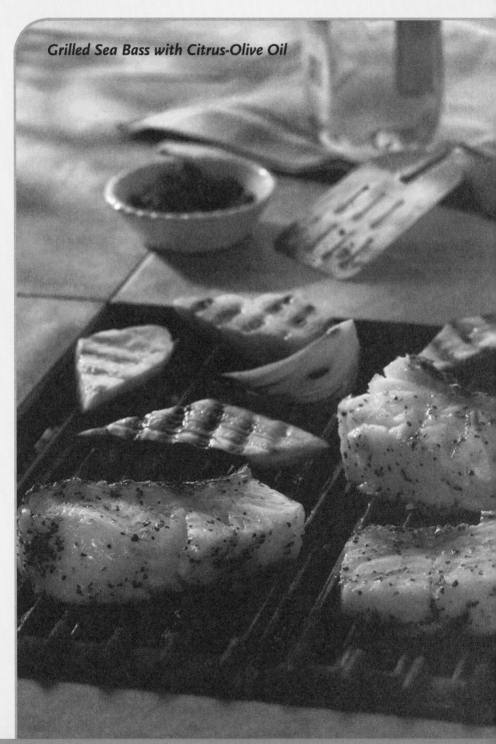

Grilled Sea Bass with Citrus-Olive Oil

Grilled Sea Bass with Citrus-Olive Oil

PREP: 10 min CHILL: 30 min GRILL: 13 min
4 servings

Ingredients
Citrus-Olive Oil (below)
1 pound sea bass, tuna or halibut fillets, about 1 inch thick
1 tablespoon canola or soybean oil
1/4 teaspoon salt
1/8 teaspoon pepper

1   Make Citrus-Olive Oil. Refrigerate 30 minutes. Heat coals
    or gas grill for direct heat. Brush all surfaces of fish with oil;
    sprinkle with salt and pepper.

2   Cover and grill fish 4 to 5 inches from medium heat 10 to
    13 minutes, turning fish after 5 minutes, until fish flakes easily
    with fork. Serve with Citrus-Olive Oil.

Citrus-Olive Oil
1 tablespoon finely chopped Kalamata olives
2 teaspoons chopped fresh parsley
1/4 teaspoon grated orange peel
1 tablespoon canola or soybean oil
1/2 teaspoon balsamic vinegar

Mix all ingredients in small bowl.

1 Serving:

Calories 180
(Calories from Fat 90)
Fat 10g
Saturated Fat 2g
(5% of Calories from
Saturated Fat)
Trans Fat 0g
Cholesterol 55mg
Omega-3 1g
Sodium 230mg

Exchanges:
3 Lean Meat, 1/2 Fat

3 Carbohydrate Choices

Carbohydrate Counting

Carbohydrates — found in breads, rice, pasta, fruits, milk, and cereals — affect blood sugar more than any other foods. Your body needs carbohydrates at all meals.

Dietitians, certified diabetes educators, and the American Diabetes Association recommend carbohydrate counting (a meal-planning technique) to provide a variety of food choices within your diabetes meal plan. On a food label, 15 grams of Total Carbohydrate equals 1 Carbohydrate Choice. For better blood-sugar control, stay consistent by eating 3 meals, similar in size, at the same times each day. Ask your doctor or dietitian about an individualized carbohydrate-counting meal plan.

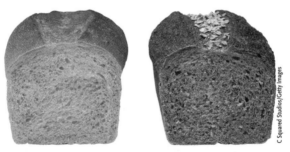

C Squared Studios/Getty Images

Whole grain bread provides a healthier carbohydrate choice versus white bread.

Notes

MONDAY

Minutes of exercise _____
Weight _____
Blood pressure _____

TUESDAY

Minutes of exercise _____
Weight _____
Blood pressure _____

WEDNESDAY

Minutes of exercise _____
Weight _____
Blood pressure _____

THURSDAY

Minutes of exercise _____
Weight _____
Blood pressure _____

FRIDAY

Minutes of exercise _____
Weight _____
Blood pressure _____

SATURDAY

Minutes of exercise _____
Weight _____
Blood pressure _____

SUNDAY

Minutes of exercise _____
Weight _____
Blood pressure _____

Things to do for next week:

Check next week's supply of:
○ blood pressure medication
○ cholesterol medication
○ aspirin
○ vitamins
○ diabetes medication
○ lancets
○ glucose test strips

Fresh Spinach, Orange and Red Onion Salad

1 Serving:

Calories 265
(Calories from Fat 35)
Fat 4g
Saturated Fat 2g
(6% of Calories from
Saturated Fat)
Trans Fat 0g
Cholesterol 20mg
Omega-3 0g
Sodium 895mg

Exchanges:
2 Starch, 2 1/2 Very
Lean Meat, 1/2 Fat

PREP: 15 min   BROIL: 5 min
8 servings

Ingredients
4 medium seedless oranges
Orange juice
1/3 cup honey
3 tablespoons raspberry vinegar
2 tablespoons canola or soybean oil
1/2 teaspoon salt
1 medium red onion, cut into 1/4-inch-thick slices
8 cups torn washed fresh spinach leaves (from
    10-ounce bag), stems removed

1   Arrange spinach on serving platter or
    individual serving plates.

2   Peel off eight 2 1/2 x 2-inch strips of orange
    peel with vegetable peeler, being careful to
remove only orange part. Cut strips lengthwise into thin slivers.

3   Cut remaining peel and white pith from oranges with sharp
    knife. Remove segments of orange by cutting between
    membranes, catching juice in small bowl; set orange
    segments aside. Squeeze membranes of oranges into bowl
    to remove all of juice; if necessary, add orange juice to make
    1/2 cup. Beat in honey, vinegar, oil and salt with wire whisk.

4   Place onion slices in single layer on ungreased cookie sheet;
    brush with orange juice mixture. Broil 2 to 3 inches from heat
    4 to 5 minutes or just until edges begin to darken.

5   Arrange orange segments on spinach. Separate onion slices
    into rings; scatter over oranges. Drizzle with remaining
    orange juice mixture; garnish with strips of orange peel.

1.5 Carbohydrate Choices

Double-Chocolate Chip Cookies

PREP: 30 min   BAKE: 8 to 9 min per sheet
2 dozen cookies

Ingredients
1/2 cup packed brown sugar
1/4 cup butter softened
1/2 teaspoon vanilla
1 egg white
1 cup all-purpose flour
3 tablespoons baking cocoa
1/2 cup semisweet chocolate chips
1/8 teaspoon salt
1/2 cup semisweet chocolate chips

1   Heat oven to 375°. Beat brown sugar and butter in large bowl with electric mixer on medium speed until light and fluffy, or mix with spoon. Beat in vanilla and egg white.

2   Stir in flour, cocoa, baking soda and salt. Stir in chocolate chips. Drop dough by teaspoonfuls about 2 inches apart onto ungreased cookie sheet.

3   Bake 8 to 9 minutes or until set (do not overbake). Cool 1 minute; remove from cookie sheet to wire rack.

1 Serving:

Calories 75
(Calories from Fat 25)
Fat 3g
Saturated Fat 2g
(23% of Calories from Saturated Fat)
Trans Fat 0g
Cholesterol 5mg
Omega-3 0g
Sodium 60mg

Exchanges:
1 Other Carbohydrates,
1/2 Fat

1 Carbohydrate Choice

Stress Management

Stress without relief can damage your health. To protect your health, treat yourself each day to many brief periods of relaxation, joy, or healthy pleasure. There are many ways to do this. Take a deep breath and relax for a minute while you have a pleasant thought. Laugh! Give a loved one a hug. Take a warm, relaxed bath. Try meditation. Exercise regularly. Listen to soothing music. All of these help manage the effects of stress.

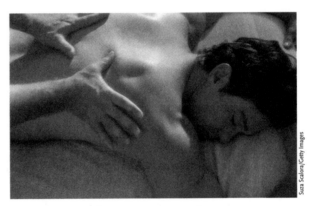

Try a massage as part of a stress management routine.

Gray skies are just clouds passing over.
—Duke Ellington

Notes

MONDAY

Minutes of exercise _____
Weight _____
Blood pressure _____

TUESDAY

Minutes of exercise _____
Weight _____
Blood pressure _____

WEDNESDAY

Minutes of exercise _____
Weight _____
Blood pressure _____

THURSDAY

Minutes of exercise _____
Weight _____
Blood pressure _____

FRIDAY

Minutes of exercise _____
Weight _____
Blood pressure _____

SATURDAY

Minutes of exercise _____
Weight _____
Blood pressure _____

SUNDAY

Minutes of exercise _____
Weight _____
Blood pressure _____

Things to do for next week:

Check next week's supply of:
- ○ blood pressure medication
- ○ cholesterol medication
- ○ aspirin
- ○ vitamins
- ○ diabetes medication
- ○ lancets
- ○ glucose test strips

Molasses Lover's Carrot-Raisin Cookies

PREP: 20 min   BAKE: 6 to 9 min per sheet   COOL: 30 min
About 3 dozen cookies

Ingredients
2/3 cup dark molasses
1/2 cup canola or soybean oil
1 egg
1 cup all-purpose flour
1 cup plus 2 tablespoons ground flaxseed or flaxseed meal
1/2 cup wheat germ
1/2 teaspoon baking powder
1/2 teaspoon baking soda
1 cup shredded carrots
1/2 cup golden raisins Glaze (below)

1   Heat oven to 375°. Mix molasses, oil and egg in medium bowl. Stir in remaining ingredients. Drop dough by tablespoonfuls onto ungreased cookie sheet.

2   Bake 6 to 9 minutes or just until set. Let stand 1 minute; remove from cookie sheet to wire rack. Cool completely, about 30 minutes. Make Glaze; drizzle about 1/2 teaspoon over each cookie.

Glaze
1 cup powdered sugar
4 to 5 teaspoons fat-free (skim) milk
1/2 teaspoon vanilla

Mix ingredients in small bowl until smooth.

1 Cookie:

Calories 110
(Calories from Fat 45)
Fat 5g
Saturated Fat 0g
(4% of Calories from Saturated Fat)
Trans Fat 0g
Cholesterol 5mg
Omega-3 1g
Sodium 30mg

Exchanges:
1 Other Carbohydrates,
1 Fat

1 Carbohydrate Choice

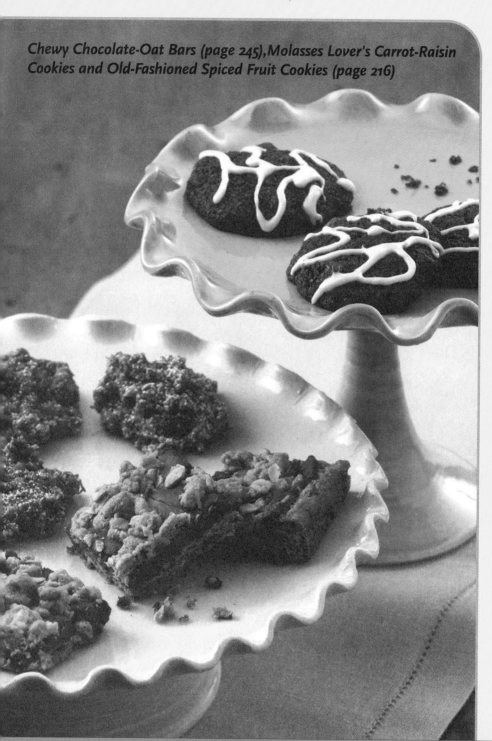

Chewy Chocolate-Oat Bars (page 245), Molasses Lover's Carrot-Raisin Cookies and Old-Fashioned Spiced Fruit Cookies (page 216)

Flu Season

Depending on the severity of your condition, heart disease can make your immune system more vulnerable to severe complications from the flu and pneumonia. People with heart disease should get a flu shot before the flu season, which generally runs November through March. Check with your doctor about this vaccination. The shot will not only protect you from the flu, but it can also help you avoid passing the flu on to your loved ones.

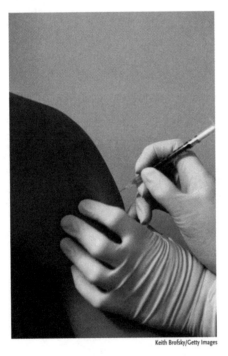

Keith Brofsky/Getty Images

Check with your doctor to see if you should receive a flu shot each fall.

Success isn't measured by the position you reach in life; it's measured by the obstacles you overcome.
—Booker T. Washington

Notes

MONDAY

Minutes of exercise _____
Weight _____
Blood pressure _____

TUESDAY

Minutes of exercise _____
Weight _____
Blood pressure _____

WEDNESDAY

Minutes of exercise _____
Weight _____
Blood pressure _____

THURSDAY

Minutes of exercise _____
Weight _____
Blood pressure _____

FRIDAY

Minutes of exercise _____
Weight _____
Blood pressure _____

SATURDAY

Minutes of exercise _____
Weight _____
Blood pressure _____

SUNDAY

Minutes of exercise _____
Weight _____
Blood pressure _____

Things to do for next week:

Check next week's supply of:
○ blood pressure medication
○ cholesterol medication
○ aspirin
○ vitamins
○ diabetes medication
○ lancets
○ glucose test strips

Old-Fashioned Spiced Fruit Cookies

PREP: 20 min BAKE: 10 to 12 min per sheet
About 3 dozen cookies

Ingredients
1 medium tart red apple, unpeeled, cored and cut into wedges
1 medium orange, unpeeled and cut into wedges
1 cup chopped dates
3/4 cup packed brown sugar
1/2 cup canola or soybean oil
1 egg
1 cup all-purpose flour
1 cup whole wheat flour
1 cup plus 2 tablespoons ground flaxseed or flaxseed meal
1 teaspoon baking soda
1 teaspoon ground cinnamon
1/4 teaspoon salt
1/4 teaspoon ground nutmeg
1/4 teaspoon ground cloves

1 Heat oven to 350°. Place apple, orange and dates in blender or food processor. Cover and blend or process until well blended.

2 Mix brown sugar, oil and egg in large bowl. Stir in remaining ingredients and fruit mixture. Drop dough by tablespoonfuls onto ungreased cookie sheet.

3 Bake 10 to 12 minutes or until light golden brown. Immediately remove from cookie sheet.

2 Cookies:

Calories 220
(Calories from Fat 80)
Fat 9g
Saturated Fat 1 g
(2% of Calories from
Saturated Fat)
Trans Fat 0g
Cholesterol 10mg
Omega-3 2g
Sodium 115mg

Exchanges:
1 Starch, 1 Other
Carbohydrates, 2 Fat

2 Carbohydrate Choices

Guacamole and Chips

PREP: 20 min CHILL: 1 hr
11 servings (1/4 cup dip with 5 tortilla chips each)

Ingredients
2 jalapeño chilies*
2 ripe large avocados
2 tablespoons lime or lemon juice
2 tablespoons finely chopped fresh cilantro
1/2 teaspoon salt
Dash of pepper
1 clove garlic, finely chopped
2 medium tomatoes, finely chopped (1 1/2 cups)
1 medium onion, chopped (1/2 cup)
1/2 bag (13 1/2 ounces) baked tortilla chips

*2 tablespoons canned chopped green chiles can be substituted for the
jalapeño chilies.

1 Remove stems, seeds and membranes
from chilies; chop chilies. Cut avocados
lengthwise in half; remove pit and peel.
Place avocados in medium glass or
plastic bowl; mash.

2 Stir in chilies and remaining ingredients
except tortilla chips. Cover and refrigerate
at least 1 hour to blend flavors. Serve with
tortilla chips.

1/2 Cup:

Calories 135
(Calories from Fat 45)
Fat 5g
Saturated Fat 1g
(6% of Calories from
Saturated Fat)
Trans Fat 0g
Cholesterol 0mg
Omega-3 0g
Sodium 240mg

Exchanges:
1 Starch, 1 Fat

1 Carbohydrate Choice

Dental Care

Prevention is the key to good dental health.

- Control blood sugar. Good control can help prevent periodontal (gum) disease.
- Brush and floss every day. Check for bleeding, dryness, soreness, white patches, or a bad taste. All of these are reasons to visit your dentist.
- Visit your dentist at least every 6 months. Be sure to tell your dentist if you have diabetes.
- Quit smoking. Smoking makes gum disease worse.

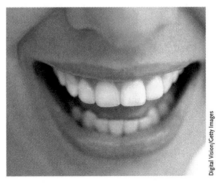

Visit your dentist every 6 months.

Notes

MONDAY

Minutes of exercise _____
Weight _____
Blood pressure _____

TUESDAY

Minutes of exercise _____
Weight _____
Blood pressure _____

WEDNESDAY

Minutes of exercise _____
Weight _____
Blood pressure _____

THURSDAY

Minutes of exercise _____
Weight _____
Blood pressure _____

FRIDAY

Minutes of exercise _____
Weight _____
Blood pressure _____

SATURDAY

Minutes of exercise _____
Weight _____
Blood pressure _____

SUNDAY

Minutes of exercise _____
Weight _____
Blood pressure _____

Things to do for next week:

Check next week's supply of:

- ○ blood pressure medication
- ○ cholesterol medication
- ○ aspirin
- ○ vitamins
- ○ diabetes medication
- ○ lancets
- ○ glucose test strips

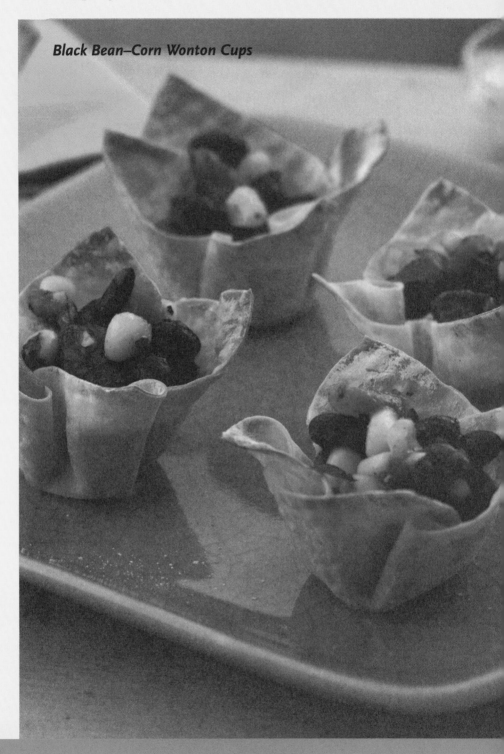

Black Bean–Corn Wonton Cups

Black Bean–Corn Wonton Cups

PREP: 25 min BAKE: 10 min
36 appetizers

Ingredients
36 wonton wrappers (3 1/2-inch squares)
2/3 cup chunky-style salsa
1/4 cup chopped fresh cilantro
1/2 teaspoon ground cumin
1/2 teaspoon chili powder
1 can (15 1/4 ounces) whole kernel corn, drained
1 can (15 ounces) black beans, rinsed and drained
1/4 cup plus 2 tablespoons fat-free sour cream

1 Heat oven to 350°. Gently fit 1 wonton wrapper into each of
   36 small muffin cups, 1 3/4 x 1 inch. Bake 8 to 10 minutes or
   until light golden brown. Remove from pan; cool on wire
   racks.

2 Mix remaining ingredients except sour
   cream in medium bowl. Just before serving,
   spoon bean mixture into wonton cups.
   Top each with 1/2 teaspoon sour cream.

1 Serving:
Calories 45
(Calories from Fat 0)
Fat 0g
Saturated Fat 0g
(1% of Calories from
Saturated Fat)
Trans Fat 0g
Cholesterol 5mg
Omega-3 0g
Sodium 100mg

Exchanges:
1/2 Starch

3 Carbohydrate Choices

Vitamin D

Vitamin D is important in your diet. The recommended daily allowance for vitamin D is 400 I.U. (one 8-ounce glass of milk equals 100 I.U. of vitamin D). Proper amounts can be obtained through food sources — dairy products, leafy greens, yogurt, nuts, whole grains, broccoli, or salmon — or supplements.

Vitamin D, which helps the body absorb calcium, is made when the skin absorbs sunlight and combines it with a form of cholesterol. While excessive sun exposure is harmful, 30 minutes of natural, outdoor sunlight per day is effective in producing sufficient amounts of vitamin D.

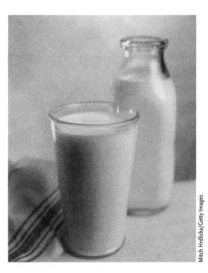

Milk is a good source of vitamin D.

Mitch Hrdlicka/Getty Images

Character may be manifested in the great moments, but it is made in the small ones.
—Phillips Brooks

Notes

MONDAY

Minutes of exercise _____
Weight _____
Blood pressure _____

TUESDAY

Minutes of exercise _____
Weight _____
Blood pressure _____

WEDNESDAY

Minutes of exercise _____
Weight _____
Blood pressure _____

THURSDAY

Minutes of exercise _____
Weight _____
Blood pressure _____

FRIDAY

Minutes of exercise _____
Weight _____
Blood pressure _____

SATURDAY

Minutes of exercise _____
Weight _____
Blood pressure _____

SUNDAY

Minutes of exercise _____
Weight _____
Blood pressure _____

Things to do for next week:

Check next week's supply of:
- ○ blood pressure medication
- ○ cholesterol medication
- ○ aspirin
- ○ vitamins
- ○ diabetes medication
- ○ lancets
- ○ glucose test strips

Shrimp Florentine Stir-Fry

PREP: 10 min COOK: 7 min
4 servings

Ingredients
1 tablespoon canola or soybean oil
1 pound uncooked peeled deveined medium shrimp, thawed if frozen
4 cups lightly packed washed spinach leaves
1 can (14 ounces) baby corn nuggets, drained
1/4 cup coarsely chopped drained roasted red bell peppers (from 7-ounce jar)
1 1/2 teaspoons chopped fresh or 1/2 teaspoon dried tarragon leaves
1/2 teaspoon garlic salt
Lemon wedges

1   Heat wok or 12-inch nonstick skillet over medium-high heat.
    Add oil; rotate wok to coat side.

2   Add shrimp; stir-fry 2 to 3 minutes or until shrimp are pink
    and firm. Add spinach, corn, bell peppers, tarragon and garlic
    salt; stir-fry 2 to 4 minutes or until spinach is wilted. Serve
    with lemon wedges.

1 Serving:

Calories 210
(Calories from Fat 45)
Fat 5g
Saturated Fat 1g
(3% of Calories from
Saturated Fat)
Trans Fat 0g
Cholesterol 160mg
Omega-3 1g
Sodium 540mg

Exchanges:
4 Vegetable,
2 Lean Meat

1 Carbohydrate Choice

Caribbean Swordfish with Papaya Salsa

PREP: 10 min MARINATE: 2 hr BROIL: 16 min
4 servings

Ingredients
Papaya Salsa (below)
1 tablespoon grated lime peel
1/4 cup grapefruit juice
1/2 teaspoon salt
4 swordfish or shark steaks, 1 inch thick (about 1 1/2 pounds)

1 clove garlic, finely chopped
1/4 cup lime juice

1 Place fish in ungreased square baking dish, 8 x 8 x 2 inches. Mix remaining ingredients except Papaya Salsa in small bowl; pour over fish. Cover and refrigerate 2 hours. Make Papaya Salsa.

2 Set oven control to broil. Spray broiler pan rack with cooking spray. Remove fish from marinade; reserve marinade. Place fish on rack in broiler pan.

3 Broil with tops about 4 inches from heat about 16 minutes, turning and brushing with marinade after 8 minutes, until fish flakes easily with fork. Discard any remaining marinade. Serve fish with salsa.

Papaya Salsa
1 large papaya, peeled, seeded and chopped (2 cups)
1/4 cup finely chopped red bell pepper
1 medium green onion, finely chopped (1 tablespoon)
1 tablespoon chopped fresh cilantro
2 to 3 tablespoons grapefruit juice
1/8 teaspoon salt

Mix all ingredients in glass or plastic bowl. Cover and refrigerate 1 hour.

1 Serving:
Calories 245
(Calories from Fat 70)
Fat 8g
Saturated Fat 2g
(8% of Calories from Saturated Fat)
Trans Fat 0g
Cholesterol 90mg
Omega-3 2g
Sodium 460mg

Exchanges:
1 Fruit, 4 Very Lean Meat, 1 Fat

1 Carbohydrate Choice

Food Labels

The U.S. Food and Drug Administration (FDA) regulates food labeling, which provides precise, comprehensive nutrition information for almost every food item sold in stores. Words such as "light," "low fat," "sugar free," and "reduced" all have standardized definitions.

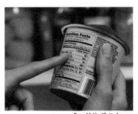

Talk to a registered dietitian about how to read food labels properly.

Ryan McVay/Getty Images

Important information found on food labels is:

- Number of calories as well as grams of fat, fiber, carbohydrates, and milligrams of cholesterol
- Serving size information given in measurements such as cups, tablespoons, and ounces

Mistakes are their own instructors.
—Horace

Notes

MONDAY

Minutes of exercise _____
Weight _____
Blood pressure _____

TUESDAY

Minutes of exercise _____
Weight _____
Blood pressure _____

WEDNESDAY

Minutes of exercise _____
Weight _____
Blood pressure _____

THURSDAY

Minutes of exercise _____
Weight _____
Blood pressure _____

FRIDAY

Minutes of exercise _____
Weight _____
Blood pressure _____

SATURDAY

Minutes of exercise _____
Weight _____
Blood pressure _____

SUNDAY

Minutes of exercise _____
Weight _____
Blood pressure _____

Things to do for next week:

Check next week's supply of:
○ vitamins
○ blood pressure medication   ○ diabetes medication
○ cholesterol medication   ○ lancets
○ aspirin   ○ glucose test strips

Apple-Rosemary Pork and Barley

PREP: 15 min   COOK: 18 min
4 servings

Ingredients
1 1/2 cups apple juice
3/4 cup uncooked quick-cooking barley
2 tablespoons chopped fresh or 2 teaspoons dried rosemary leaves, crushed
3/4-pound pork tenderloin
2 teaspoons canola or soybean oil
1 medium onion, chopped (1/2 cup)
1 clove garlic, finely chopped
1/4 cup apple jelly
1 large unpeeled red cooking apple, sliced (1 1/2 cups)

1   Heat apple juice to boiling in 2-quart saucepan. Stir in barley and 1 tablespoon of the rosemary; reduce heat to low. Cover and simmer 10 to 12 minutes until liquid is absorbed and barley is tender.

2   While barley is cooking, cut pork into 1/4-inch slices.

3   Heat oil in 10-inch nonstick skillet over medium-high heat. Cook pork, onion, garlic and remaining 1 tablespoon rosemary in hot oil about 5 minutes, stirring frequently, until pork is no longer pink in center. Stir in apple jelly and apple slices; cook until hot. Serve over barley.

2.5 Carbohydrate Choices

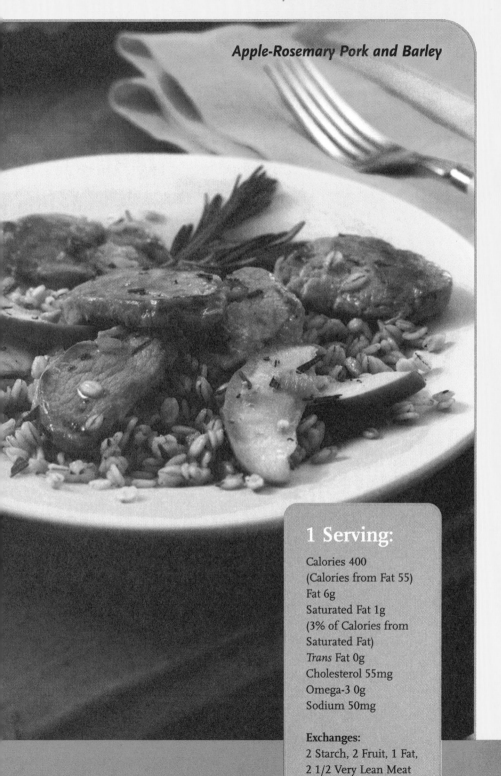

Apple-Rosemary Pork and Barley

1 Serving:

Calories 400
(Calories from Fat 55)
Fat 6g
Saturated Fat 1g
(3% of Calories from
Saturated Fat)
Trans Fat 0g
Cholesterol 55mg
Omega-3 0g
Sodium 50mg

Exchanges:
2 Starch, 2 Fruit, 1 Fat,
2 1/2 Very Lean Meat

Artificial Sweeteners

For individuals who have diabetes, replacing table sugar with an artificial sweetener can provide that sweet flavor without adding extra carbohydrates and calories or raising your blood-sugar level. There are many types of artificial sweeteners on the market today to help limit sugar intake.

The FDA has approved the use of these sweeteners and concludes that they are safe for human consumption.

Artificial sweeteners currently available on the market are:

• Saccharin — can be used in hot or cold foods
• Aspartame (NutraSweet®) — not recommended for baking
• Acesulfame potassium (Sweet One®) — can be used in baking and cooking
• Sucralose (Splenda®) — a no-calorie sweetener derived from sugar; can be used anywhere sugar is used

Notes

MONDAY

Minutes of exercise _____
Weight _____
Blood pressure _____

TUESDAY

Minutes of exercise _____
Weight _____
Blood pressure _____

WEDNESDAY

Minutes of exercise _____
Weight _____
Blood pressure _____

THURSDAY

Minutes of exercise _____
Weight _____
Blood pressure _____

FRIDAY

Minutes of exercise _____
Weight _____
Blood pressure _____

SATURDAY

Minutes of exercise _____
Weight _____
Blood pressure _____

SUNDAY

Minutes of exercise _____
Weight _____
Blood pressure _____

Things to do for next week:

Check next week's supply of:

- ○ blood pressure medication
- ○ cholesterol medication
- ○ aspirin
- ○ vitamins
- ○ diabetes medication
- ○ lancets
- ○ glucose test strips

Snap Pea Frittata

PREP: 5 min COOK: 10 min BROIL: 2 min
6 servings

Ingredients
1 tablespoon olive or canola oil
1/2 cup sliced onion
1 teaspoon dried tarragon leaves
1 package (9 ounces) frozen sugar snap peas in a pouch, thawed
1 cup shredded lettuce
6 eggs
1/2 teaspoon salt
1/4 teaspoon pepper
2 tablespoons grated Parmesan cheese

1 Set oven control to broil. Heat oil in 10-inch ovenproof skillet over medium heat. Cook onion in oil 2 minutes, stirring frequently. Stir in tarragon and sugar snap peas; cook uncovered 3 minutes, stirring frequently, until peas are tender. Stir in lettuce.

2 Beat eggs with salt and pepper in medium bowl with wire whisk. Pour over vegetables in skillet. Cook 8 to 10 minutes or until eggs just begin to set.

3 Sprinkle with cheese. Broil 5 inches from heat 1 to 2 minutes or until frittata is golden brown and puffs up.

1 Serving:

Calories 125
(Calories from Fat 70)
Fat 8g
Saturated Fat 2g
(17% of Calories from Saturated Fat)
Trans Fat 0g
Cholesterol 215mg
Omega-3 0g
Sodium 300mg

Exchanges:
1 Vegetable,
1 Medium-Fat Meat

0 Carbohydrate Choices

Harvest Salad

PREP: 15 min COOK: 12 min STAND: 5 min COOL: 30 min
6 servings

Ingredients
1 1/3 cups water
2/3 cup uncooked quick-cooking barley
2 cups frozen whole kernel corn, thawed
1/2 cup dried cranberries
1/4 cup thinly sliced green onions (4 medium)
1 medium unpeeled apple, chopped (about 1 cup)
1 small carrot, coarsely shredded (about 1/3 cup)
2 tablespoons canola or soybean oil
2 tablespoons honey
1 tablespoon lemon juice

1 Serving:

Calories 360
(Calories from Fat 55)
Fat 6g
Saturated Fat 1g
(1% of Calories from
Saturated Fat)
Trans Fat 0g
Cholesterol 0mg
Omega-3 0g
Sodium 15mg

Exchanges:
3 Starch, 1 Fruit,
1 Other Carbohydrates

1 Heat water to boiling in 1 1/2-quart saucepan. Stir in barley; reduce heat to low. Cover and simmer 10 to 12 minutes or until tender. Let stand covered 5 minutes. Uncover; cool 30 minutes.

2 Mix barley, corn, cranberries, green onions, apple and carrot in large bowl.

3 Shake oil, honey and lemon juice in tightly covered container. Pour over barley mixture; toss to mix.

3 Carbohydrate Choices

Bonus Recipe Section

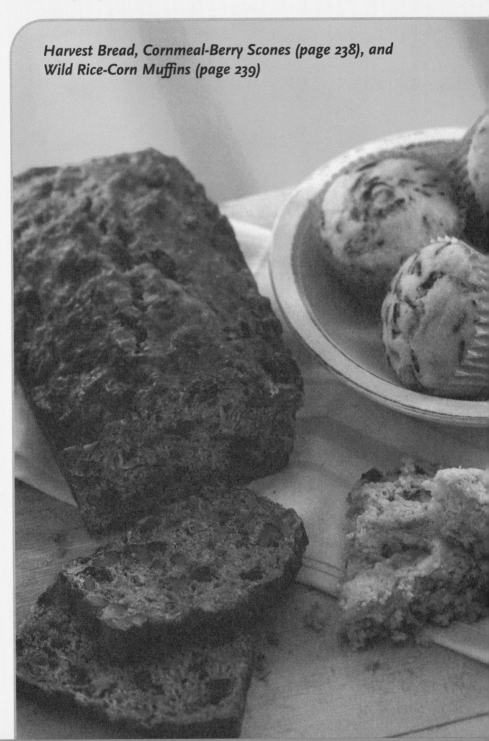

Harvest Bread, Cornmeal-Berry Scones (page 238), and Wild Rice-Corn Muffins (page 239)

Harvest Bread

PREP: 15 min   BAKE: 55 min   COOL: 1 hr 10 min
1 loaf (16 slices)

Ingredients
1 can (8 ounces) crushed pineapple in juice, drained and
   juice reserved
1/4 cup fat-free cholesterol-free egg product or 1 egg
2 tablespoons canola or soybean oil
1 1/2 cups all-purpose flour
3/4 cup packed brown sugar
1/2 cup raisins
1 teaspoon baking powder
1/2 teaspoon baking soda
1/2 teaspoon salt
1/2 teaspoon ground cinnamon
1 cup shredded carrots (1 1/2 medium)
1 cup walnuts, chopped

1 Serving:

Calories 185
(Calories from Fat 65)
Fat 7g
Saturated Fat 1g
(3% of Calories from
Saturated Fat)
Trans Fat 0g
Cholesterol 0mg
Omega-3 1g
Sodium 160mg

Exchanges:
1 Starch, 1 Other
Carbohydrates, 1 Fat

1   Heat oven to 350°. Spray loaf pan,
    8 1/2 x 4 1/2 x 2 1/2 inches, with cooking
    spray. Discard 3 tablespoons of the
    pineapple juice. Mix remaining juice, pineapple, egg product
    and oil in medium bowl. Stir in remaining ingredients until
    blended. Spread batter in pan.

2   Bake 50 to 55 minutes or until toothpick inserted in center
    comes out clean. Cool 10 minutes. Remove from pan to wire
    rack. Cool completely, about 1 hour, before slicing.

3 Carbohydrate Choices

Cornmeal-Berry Scones

....

PREP: 15 min BAKE: 15 min
12 scones

Ingredients

1 cup whole-grain yellow cornmeal
2 teaspoons baking powder
1 tablespoon vanilla soy milk
1/4 teaspoon grated orange or lemon peel
6 tablespoons firm butter, cut into cubes
1 1/2 cups strawberries, coarsely chopped*

2 tablespoons sugar
1 cup all-purpose flour
1 to 2 tablespoons sugar
1/4 teaspoon salt
1/2 cup vanilla soy milk
1/2 teaspoon baking soda

*1 1/2 cups frozen strawberries, thawed, drained and coarsely chopped, can be substituted. Toss with an additional 1/4 cup flour before adding to batter.

1   Heat oven to 425°. Spray cookie sheet with cooking spray, or line with cooking parchment paper.

2   Mix flour, cornmeal, 2 tablespoons sugar, the baking powder, baking soda, orange peel and salt in large bowl. Cut in butter using pastry blender, just until mixture looks like coarse crumbs. Stir in 1/2 cup soy milk and the orange juice just until flour is moistened. Fold in strawberries.

3   Place dough on floured surface. Knead 6 to 8 times to form a ball. Divide in half; shape into two 6 x 1/2-inch rounds on cookie sheet. Brush rounds with 1 tablespoon soy milk and sprinkle with 1 to 2 tablespoons sugar. Cut each round into 6 wedges.

4   Bake 12 to 15 minutes or until tops are lightly browned. Separate wedges; serve warm.

1 Serving:

Calories 150
(Calories from Fat 55)
Fat 6g
Saturated Fat 4g
(21% of Calories from
Saturated Fat)
Trans Fat 0g
Cholesterol 15mg
Omega-3 0g
Sodium 230mg

Exchanges:
1 Starch, 1/2 Fruit,
1 Fat

1.5 Carbohydrate Choices

Wild Rice–Corn Muffins

PREP: 10 min   BAKE: 25 min
12 muffins

Ingredients
3/4 cup fat-free (skim) milk
1/4 cup canola or soybean oil
1/4 cup fat-free cholesterol-free egg product,
   2 egg whites or 1 egg
1 cup all-purpose flour
1/2 cup sugar
1/2 cup whole-grain yellow cornmeal
2 1/2 teaspoons baking powder
1/4 teaspoon salt
3/4 cup cooked wild rice
1/2 cup chopped fresh or frozen cranberries

1 Muffin:

Calories 155
(Calories from Fat 45)
Fat 5g
Saturated Fat 0g
(2% of Calories from
Saturated Fat)
Trans Fat 0g
Cholesterol 0mg
Omega-3 0g
Sodium 170mg

Exchanges:
1 Fat, 1 Starch, 1/2
Other Carbohydrates

1   Heat oven to 400°. Spray 12 medium muffin cups,
2 1/2 x 1 1/4 inches, with cooking spray, or line with paper
baking cups. Mix milk, oil and egg product in large bowl.

2   Stir in flour, sugar, cornmeal, baking powder and salt all
at once just until flour is moistened. Fold in wild rice and
cranberries. Divide batter evenly among muffin cups.

3   Bake 20 to 25 minutes or until golden brown. Immediately
remove from pan. Serve warm.

1.5 Carbohydrate Choices

Broiled Dijon Burgers

PREP: 10 min BROIL: 12 min
6 servings

Ingredients
1/4 cup fat-free cholesterol-free egg product or 2 egg whites
2 tablespoons fat-free (skim) milk
2 teaspoons Dijon mustard or horseradish sauce
1/4 teaspoon salt
1/8 teaspoon pepper
1 cup soft bread crumbs (about 2 slices bread)
1 small onion, finely chopped (1/4 cup)
1 pound extra-lean ground beef
6 whole-grain hamburger buns, split and toasted

1   Set oven control to broil. Spray broiler pan rack with cooking
    spray.

2   Mix egg product, milk, mustard, salt and pepper in medium
    bowl. Stir in bread crumbs and onion. Stir in beef. Shape
    mixture into 6 patties, each about 1/2 inch thick. Place patties
    on rack in broiler pan.

3   Broil with tops of patties about
    5 inches from heat 6 minutes.
    Turn; broil until meat
    thermometer inserted in
    center reads 160°, about 4 to
    6 minutes longer. Serve patties
    in buns.

1 Serving:

Calories 250
(Calories from Fat 55)
Fat 6g
Saturated Fat 2g
(7% of Calories from
Saturated Fat)
Trans Fat 0g
Cholesterol 45mg
Omega-3 0g
Sodium 470mg

Exchanges:
2 Starch,
2 1/2 Very Lean Meat

1.5 Carbohydrate Choices

Sweet Potato Wedges

PREP: 10 min BAKE: 30 min
4 servings

Ingredients
4 medium sweet potatoes (1 1/2 pounds), peeled and cut lengthwise
   into 1/2-inch wedges
2 tablespoons canola or soybean oil
1/2 teaspoon salt
1/4 teaspoon pepper

1   Heat oven to 450°. Brush jelly roll pan, 15 1/2 x 10 1/2 x 1 inch, with canola or soybean oil.

2   Toss potatoes with 2 tablespoons oil in large bowl. Sprinkle with salt and pepper. Spread potatoes in single layer in pan.

3   Bake uncovered 25 to 30 minutes, turning occasionally, until potatoes are golden brown and tender when pierced with fork.

1 Serving:

Calories 175
(Calories from Fat 65)
Fat 7g
Saturated Fat 1g
(3% of Calories from
Saturated Fat)
Trans Fat 0g
Cholesterol 0mg
Omega-3 0g
Sodium 310mg

Exchanges:
1 Starch, 1 Fat,
1 Other Carbohydrates

2 Carbohydrate Choices

Fajita Salad

PREP: 15 min COOK: 6 min
4 servings

Ingredients
3/4 pound boneless lean beef sirloin steak
1 tablespoon canola or soybean oil
2 medium bell peppers, cut into strips
1 small onion, thinly sliced
4 cups bite-size pieces salad greens
1/3 cup fat-free Italian dressing
1/4 cup fat-free plain yogurt

1 Cut beef across grain into bite-size strips. Heat oil in
   10-inch nonstick skillet over medium-high heat. Cook beef
   in oil about 3 minutes, stirring occasionally, until brown.
   Remove beef from skillet.

2 Cook bell peppers and onion in skillet about 3 minutes,
   stirring occasionally, until bell peppers are crisp-tender.
   Stir in beef.

3 Place salad greens on serving
   platter. Top with beef mixture.
   Mix dressing and yogurt in small
   bowl; drizzle over salad.

1 Serving:

Calories 175
(Calories from Fat 55)
Fat 6g
Saturated Fat 1g
(6% of Calories from
Saturated Fat)
Trans Fat 0g
Cholesterol 45mg
Omega-3 0g
Sodium 330mg

Exchanges
2 Vegetable,
2 Lean Meat

2.5 Carbohydrate Choices

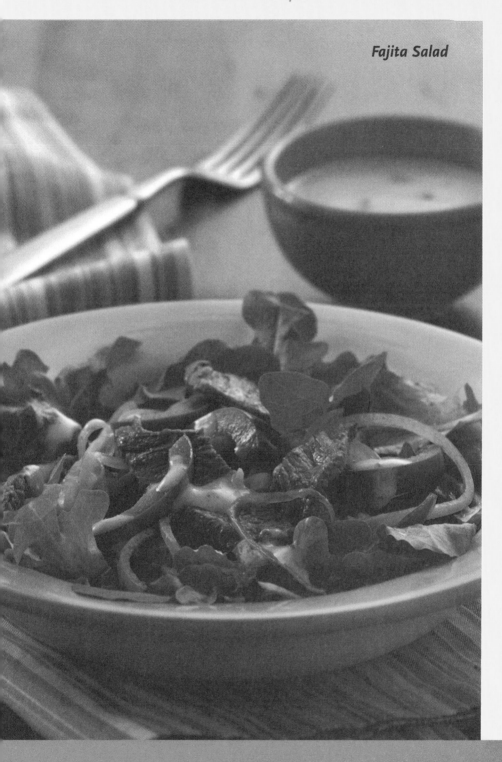

Fajita Salad

Triple-Cabbage Slaw

PREP: 15 min
4 servings

1 Serving:

Calories 50
(Calories from Fat 0)
Fat 0g
Saturated Fat 0g
(0% of Calories from
Saturated Fat)
Trans Fat 0g
Cholesterol 0mg
Omega-3 0g
Sodium 35mg

Exchanges:
1/2 Fruit, 1 Vegetable

Ingredients
2 cups thinly sliced Chinese (napa) cabbage
1 1/2 cups shredded green cabbage
1/2 cup shredded red cabbage
1 tablespoon chopped fresh chives
3 tablespoons orange marmalade
2 tablespoons rice vinegar
1 teaspoon grated gingerroot

1 Mix cabbages and chives in large glass or plastic bowl.

2 Mix marmalade, vinegar and gingerroot in small bowl until blended. Add to cabbage mixture; toss lightly to mix.

(Opposite)

1 Cookie:

Calories 165
(Calories from Fat 55)
Fat 6g
Saturated Fat 2g
(9% of Calories from
Saturated Fat)
Trans Fat 0g
Cholesterol 0mg
Omega-3 0g
Sodium 115mg

Exchanges:
1 Starch, 1 Fat,
1/2 Other Carbohydrates

1 Carbohydrate Choice≈

Chewy Chocolate-Oat Bars

PREP: 25 min BAKE: 13 min COOL: 45 min CHILL: 2 hrs
16 bars

Ingredients

1/2 cup semisweet chocolate chips
1 cup whole wheat flour
1/2 teaspoon baking soda
3/4 cup packed brown sugar
1 teaspoon vanilla
1/2 cup old-fashioned or quick-cooking oats
1/4 cup fat-free cholesterol-free egg product or 1 egg
2 tablespoons old-fashioned or quick-cooking oats
1/3 cup fat-free sweetened condensed milk (from 14-ounce can)

2 teaspoons butter, softened
1/2 teaspoon baking powder
1/4 teaspoon salt
1/4 cup canola or soybean oil

1   Heat chocolate chips and milk in 1-quart heavy saucepan over
low heat, stirring frequently, until chocolate is melted and
mixture is smooth; set aside. Heat oven to 350°. Spray square
pan, 8 x 8 x 2 or 9 x 9 x 2 inches, with cooking spray.

2   Mix flour, 1/2 cup oats, the baking powder, baking soda and
salt in large bowl; set aside. Stir brown sugar, oil, vanilla and
egg product in medium bowl with fork until smooth; stir into
flour mixture until blended. Reserve 1/2 cup dough in small
bowl for topping.

3   Pat remaining dough in pan (spray fingers with cooking spray
or lightly flour if dough is sticky). Spread chocolate mixture
over dough. Add 2 tablespoons oats and the butter to reserved
dough; mix with pastry blender or fork until crumbly. Drop
small spoonfuls of oat mixture evenly over chocolate mixture.

4   Bake 20 to 25 minutes or until top is golden and firm. Cool
completely, about 1 1/2 hours. For bars cut into 4 rows by
4 rows.

1.5 Carbohydrate Choices

Jumbo Molasses Cookies

PREP: 30 min CHILL: 3 hr BAKE: 10 to 12 min per sheet
About 3 dozen cookies

Ingredients

1 cup sugar
1 cup dark molasses
4 cups all-purpose flour
1 1/2 teaspoons ground ginger
1/2 teaspoon ground cloves
1/4 teaspoon ground allspice

1/2 cup butter, softened
1/2 cup water
1 1/2 teaspoons salt
1 teaspoon baking soda
1/2 teaspoon ground nutmeg
Sugar

1 Beat 1 cup sugar and the butter in large bowl with electric mixer on medium speed, or mix with spoon. Stir in remaining ingredients except sugar. Cover and refrigerate at least 3 hours until dough is firm.

2 Heat oven to 375°. Generously grease cookie sheet with shortening. Roll dough 1/4 inch thick on generously floured cloth-covered surface. Cut into 3-inch circles. Sprinkle with sugar. Place about 1 1/2 inches apart on cookie sheet.

3 Bake 10 to 12 minutes or until almost no indentation remains when touched lightly in center. Cool 2 minutes; remove from cookie sheet to wire rack.

1 Cookie:

Calories 125
(Calories from Fat 25)
Fat 3g
Saturated Fat 2g
(12% of Calories from Saturated Fat)
Trans Fat 0g
Cholesterol 5mg
Omega-3 0g
Sodium 150mg

Exchanges:
1/2 Starch, 1/2 Fat,
1 Other Carbohydrates

1.5 Carbohydrate Choices

Carrot-Zucchini Muffins

PREP: 10 min BAKE: 21 min
12 muffins

Ingredients
2 cups all-purpose flour
1 cup quick-cooking or old-fashioned oats
3/4 cup packed brown sugar
3 teaspoons baking powder
1/2 teaspoon cinnamon
1/4 teaspoon salt
2/3 cup fat-free (skim) milk
3 tablespoons canola or soybean oil
2 egg whites, 1/4 cup fat-free cholesterol-free egg product or 1 egg
1 cup finely shredded carrots (1 1/2 medium)
1/2 cup shredded unpeeled zucchini (1 small)

1 Heat oven to 400°. Spray 12 medium muffin cups, 2 1/2 x 1 1/4 inches, with cooking spray, or line with paper baking cups and spray paper cups with cooking spray.

2 Mix flour, oats, brown sugar, baking powder, cinnamon and salt in large bowl. Stir in milk, oil and egg whites all at once just until flour is moistened. Fold in carrots and zucchini. Divide batter evenly among muffin cups.

3 Bake 16 to 21 minutes or until golden brown and toothpick inserted in center comes out clean. Immediately remove from pan. Serve warm.

1 Cookie:

Calories 125
(Calories from Fat 25)
Fat 3g
Saturated Fat 2g
(12% of Calories from Saturated Fat)
Trans Fat 0g
Cholesterol 5mg
Omega-3 0g
Sodium 150mg

Exchanges:
1/2 Starch, 1/2 Fat,
1 Other Carbohydrates

1.5 Carbohydrate Choices

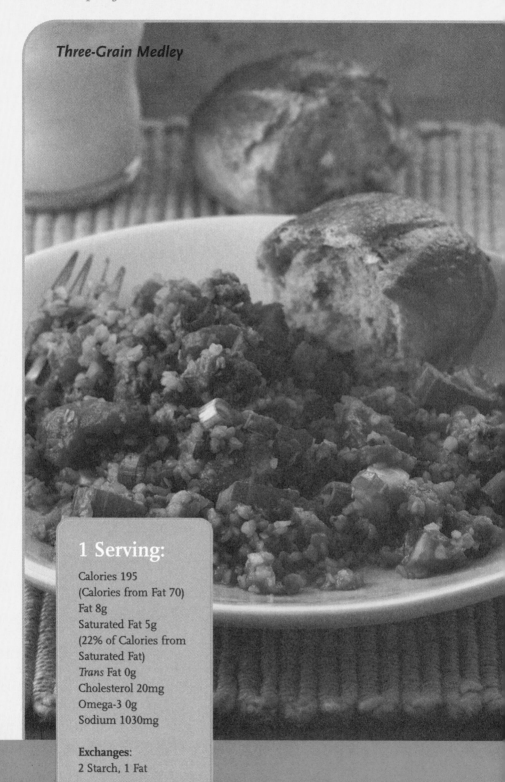

Three-Grain Medley

1 Serving:

Calories 195
(Calories from Fat 70)
Fat 8g
Saturated Fat 5g
(22% of Calories from
Saturated Fat)
Trans Fat 0g
Cholesterol 20mg
Omega-3 0g
Sodium 1030mg

Exchanges:
2 Starch, 1 Fat

Three-Grain Medley

PREP: 10 min COOK: 6 hr
6 servings

Ingredients
2/3 cup uncooked wheat berries
1/2 cup uncooked hulled or pearl barley
1/2 cup uncooked wild rice
1/4 cup chopped fresh parsley
1/4 cup butter, melted, or canola or soybean oil
2 teaspoons finely shredded lemon peel
6 medium green onions, thinly sliced (6 tablespoons)
2 cloves garlic, finely chopped
2 cans (14 ounces each) vegetable broth
1 jar (2 ounces) diced pimientos, undrained

1   Mix all ingredients in 3 1/2- to 6-quart slow cooker.

2   Cover and cook on Low heat setting 4 to 6 hours or until
    liquid is absorbed. Stir before serving.

Variation: *Use this scrumptious grain filling to stuff bell pepper
shells. Steam cleaned bell pepper halves (any color that you are in
the mood for) just until tender so that they still hold their shape.
Spoon the hot cooked grain mixture into the halves, and sprinkle
with shredded Parmesan cheese.*

3 Carbohydrate Choices

Lemon Muesli

PREP: 10 min STAND: 8 hr
3 servings (2/3 cup each)

Ingredients
1/2 cup fat-free (skim) milk
1 cup old-fashioned oats
1/2 cup lemon or orange fat-free yogurt
1 tablespoon packed brown sugar
2 tablespoons raisins or chopped dried fruit
1/2 medium banana, chopped
3 tablespoons ground flaxseed or flaxseed meal

1   Pour milk over oats in medium bowl. Let stand overnight, at least 8 hours but no longer than 12 hours.

2   Just before serving, stir in yogurt, brown sugar, raisins and banana. Spoon into individual serving bowls; sprinkle with flaxseed.

1 Serving:

Calories 215
(Calories from Fat 35)
Fat 4g
Saturated Fat 1g
(3% of Calories from
Saturated Fat)
Trans Fat 0g
Cholesterol 0mg
Omega-3 1g
Sodium 45mg

Exchanges:
1/2 Fruit, 2 1/2 Starch

3 Carbohydrate Choices

Gingered Fruit Salsa with Crispy Cinnamon Chips

PREP: 40 min BROIL: 8 min COOL: 15 min
24 servings (2 tablespoons salsa and 3 chips each)

Ingredients
1 tablespoon sugar
2 teaspoons ground cinnamon
6 flour tortillas (8 to 10 inches in diameter)
3 tablespoons canola or soybean oil
1 cup finely diced pineapple
1 cup finely diced papaya
1 cup finely diced mango
1/4 cup chopped fresh cilantro
1 tablespoon finely chopped crystallized ginger
1 tablespoon lemon juice
1/8 teaspoon salt

1 Serving:

Calories 65
(Calories from Fat 25)
Fat 3g
Saturated Fat 0g
(5% of Calories from
Saturated Fat)
Trans Fat 0g
Cholesterol 0mg
Omega-3 0g
Sodium 65mg

Exchanges:
1/2 Starch, 1/2 Fat

1 Set oven control to broil. Mix sugar and cinnamon in small bowl. Brush both sides of each tortilla with oil; sprinkle with sugar-cinnamon mixture. Cut each tortilla into 12 wedges.

2 Place tortilla wedges in single layer in 2 ungreased jelly roll pans, 15 1/2 x 10 1/2 x 1 inch, or on 2 cookie sheets. Broil 2 to 4 minutes, turning once, until crispy and golden brown. Cool completely, about 15 minutes.

3 Mix remaining ingredients in medium bowl. Serve salsa with chips.

0.5 Carbohydrate Choices

Watermelon-Kiwi-Banana Smoothie

PREP: 10 min
2 servings (1 cup each)

Ingredients
1 cup coarsely chopped seeded watermelon
1 kiwifruit, peeled and cut into pieces
1 ripe banana, frozen, peeled and cut into chunks
2 ice cubes
1/4 cup chilled apple juice

1   Place all ingredients in blender. Cover and blend on high speed about 30 seconds or until smooth.

2   Pour mixture into glasses. Serve immediately.

1 Serving:

Calories 115
(Calories from Fat 10)
Fat 1g
Saturated Fat 0g
(0% of Calories from
Saturated Fat)
Trans Fat 0g
Cholesterol 0mg
Omega-3 0g
Sodium 5mg

Exchanges:
2 Fruit

2.5 Carbohydrate Choices

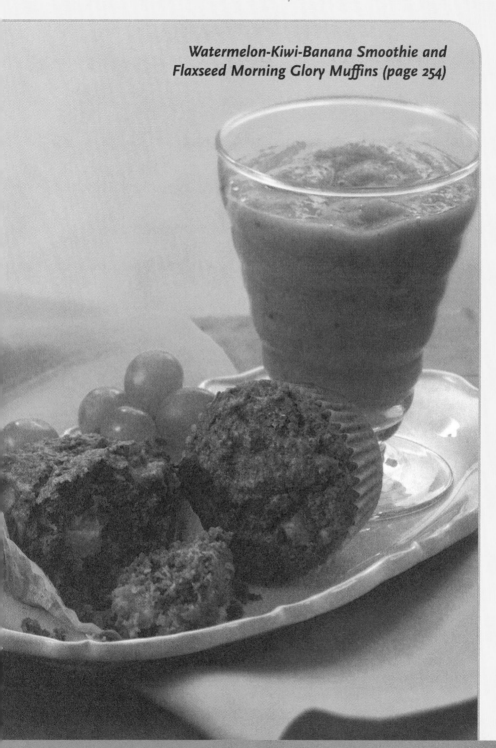

**Watermelon-Kiwi-Banana Smoothie and
Flaxseed Morning Glory Muffins (page 254)**

Flaxseed Morning Glory Muffins

PREP: 30 min BAKE: 25 min
12 muffins

Ingredients

1 cup Fiber One® cereal
1/2 cup packed brown sugar
1 cup all-purpose flour
1 tablespoon canola or soybean oil
3 teaspoons baking powder
1/2 cup finely shredded carrot
2 teaspoons ground cinnamon
3/4 cup ground flaxseed or flaxseed meal
4 egg whites or 1/2 cup fat-free cholesterol-free egg product

2/3 cup fat-free (skim) milk
1/4 cup granulated sugar
3/4 cup chopped apple
1 teaspoon vanilla
1/2 teaspoon salt
1/4 cup flaked coconut

1   Heat oven to 375°. Line 12 medium muffin cups, 2 1/2 x 1 1/4 inches, with paper baking cups and spray bottoms with nonstick baking spray.

2   Place cereal between waxed paper, plastic wrap or in plastic bag; crush with rolling pin (or crush in blender or food processor). Mix cereal and milk in large bowl; let stand about 5 minutes or until cereal is softened. Stir in remaining ingredients. Divide batter evenly among muffin cups.

3   Bake 22 to 25 minutes or until toothpick inserted in center comes out clean. Immediately remove muffins from pan. Serve warm.

1 Muffin:

Calories 160
(Calories from Fat 35)
Fat 4g
Saturated Fat 1g
(5% of Calories from Saturated Fat)
Trans Fat 0g
Cholesterol 0mg
Omega-3 1g
Sodium 280mg

Exchanges:
2 Starch

2 Carbohydrate Choices

Flank Steak Sandwiches

PREP: 10 min MARINATE: 4 hr GRILL: 12 min
6 servings

Ingredients
2 beef flank steaks (1 pound each)
1/4 cup honey
2 tablespoons soy sauce
1 tablespoon grated gingerroot
1 can or bottle (12 ounces) regular or nonalcoholic beer
8 pita breads (6 inches in diameter), cut in half to form
   pockets
2 medium tomatoes, sliced
1 large grilled sliced onion

1 Sandwich:

Calories 360
(Calories from Fat 80)
Fat 9g
Saturated Fat 3g
(8% of Calories from
Saturated Fat)
Trans Fat 0g
Cholesterol 65mg
Omega-3 0g
Sodium 510mg

Exchanges:
2 1/2 Starch,
3 Lean Meat

1 Trim fat from beef. Make cuts about 1/2 inch apart and 1/8 inch deep in diamond pattern on both sides of beef. Place in shallow glass dish. Mix honey, soy sauce, gingerroot and beer in small bowl; pour over beef. Cover and refrigerate, turning occasionally, at least 4 hours but no longer than 24 hours.

2 Brush grill rack with canola or soybean oil. Heat coals or gas grill for direct heat. Remove beef from marinade; reserve marinade. Cover and grill beef 6 inches from medium heat about 12 minutes for medium doneness, turning after 6 minutes and brushing frequently with marinade. Discard any remaining marinade.

3 Cut beef diagonally into thin slices. Serve beef in pita bread halves with tomato and onion.

2.5 Carbohydrate Choices

Barbecued Pork Tenderloin

PREP: 10 min GRILL: 22 min
6 servings

Ingredients
2 pork tenderloins (about 3/4 pound each)
1/4 teaspoon seasoned salt
1/3 cup barbecue sauce
1/4 cup teriyaki baste and glaze (from 12-ounce bottle)
2 tablespoons finely chopped onion
2 tablespoons finely chopped chipotle chili in adobo sauce (from 7-ounce can)

1 Heat coals or gas grill for direct heat. Sprinkle pork with seasoned salt. Mix remaining ingredients in small bowl. Brush pork with barbecue sauce mixture.

2 Cover and grill pork 4 to 6 inches from medium-low heat 18 to 22 minutes, turning several times and basting generously with remaining sauce mixture, until pork has slight blush of pink in center and meat thermometer inserted in center reads 160°. Discard any remaining sauce mixture.

1 Serving:

Calories 165
(Calories from Fat 35)
Fat 4g
Saturated Fat 2g
(8% of Calories from
Saturated Fat)
Trans Fat 0g
Cholesterol 70mg
Omega-3 0g
Sodium 640mg

Exchanges:
1/2 Starch,
3 1/2 Very Lean Meat

0.5 Carbohydrate Choices

Swiss Potato Patties

PREP: 10 min COOK: 43 min
8 servings

Ingredients
4 medium potatoes (1 1/3 pounds)
1 cup shredded reduced-fat Swiss cheese (4 ounces)
1/4 teaspoon salt
1/4 teaspoon pepper
1 tablespoon butter

1 Heat 1 inch water (salted if desired) to boiling in 3-quart saucepan. Add potatoes. Cover and heat to boiling; reduce heat. Simmer 30 to 35 minutes or until tender; drain.

2 Peel and shred potatoes. Mix potatoes, cheese, salt and pepper in large bowl.

3 Melt butter in 10-inch skillet over medium-high heat. Scoop half of potato mixture by 1/3 cupfuls into skillet; flatten to 1/2-inch thickness. Cook about 8 minutes, turning once, until golden brown. Repeat with remaining potato mixture.

1 Serving:

Calories 110
(Calories from Fat 45)
Fat 5g
Saturated Fat 3g
(25% of Calories from Saturated Fat)
Trans Fat 0g
Cholesterol 15mg
Omega-3 0g
Sodium 120mg

Exchanges:
1 Starch, 1/2 Fat

1 Carbohydrate Choice

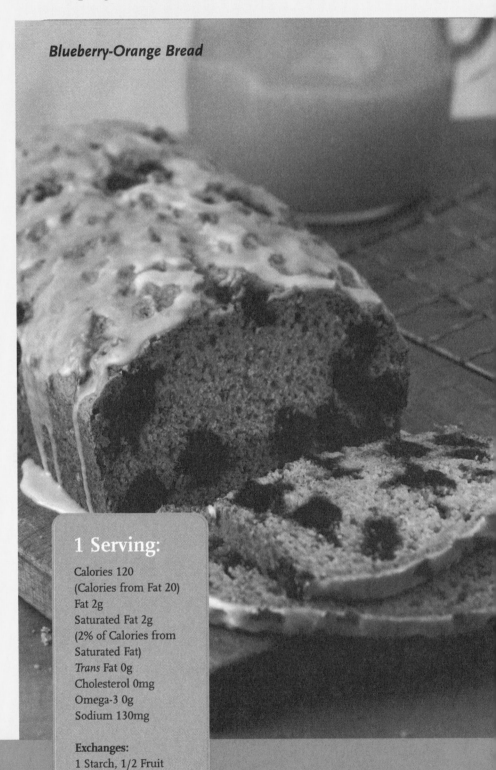

Blueberry-Orange Bread

1 Serving:

Calories 120
(Calories from Fat 20)
Fat 2g
Saturated Fat 2g
(2% of Calories from
Saturated Fat)
Trans Fat 0g
Cholesterol 0mg
Omega-3 0g
Sodium 130mg

Exchanges:
1 Starch, 1/2 Fruit

Blueberry-Orange Bread

PREP: 18 min BAKE: 60 min
1 loaf (24 slices)

Ingredients

Vanilla Glaze (below)
2 cups Total® cereal, crushed
1/4 cup orange or lemon juice
2 cups all-purpose flour
1 1/2 teaspoons baking powder
2 tablespoons canola or soybean oil
1 tablespoon grated orange or lemon peel
1 cup fresh or frozen (thawed) blueberries

3/4 cup water
1/2 teaspoon vanilla
1 cup sugar
1/2 teaspoon baking soda
1 egg
1/2 teaspoon salt

1 Heat oven to 350°. Grease bottom only of loaf pan, 9 x 5 x 3 inches, with shortening.

2 Mix cereal, water, orange peel, orange juice and vanilla in large bowl; let stand 10 minutes. Stir in remaining ingredients except blueberries and Vanilla Glaze. Gently stir in blueberries. Pour into pan.

3 Bake 50 to 60 minutes or until toothpick inserted in center comes out clean. Cool 10 minutes. Loosen sides of loaf; remove from pan to wire rack. Cool completely, about 1 hour.

4 Make Vanilla Glaze; drizzle over loaf. Wrap tightly and store at room temperature up to 4 days or refrigerate up to 10 days.

Vanilla Glaze
1/2 cup powdered sugar
1/4 teaspoon vanilla
2 to 3 teaspoons milk

Mix all ingredients until smooth and thin enough to drizzle.

3 Carbohydrate Choices

Wilted Spinach Vinaigrette

PREP: 10 min
6 servings

Ingredients
1 tablespoon canola or soybean oil
2 cloves garlic, minced
1 package (10 ounces) washed fresh spinach leaves, stems removed
1/3 cup raisins
1/4 cup sunflower nuts or pine nuts
2 teaspoons sugar
2 tablespoons white wine vinegar

1 Heat oil in 4-quart nonstick Dutch oven over medium heat. Cook garlic in oil 1 minute, stirring constantly.

2 Add spinach and raisins; cook about 1 minute, stirring constantly, or just until spinach is barely wilted. Remove from heat; stir in sunflower nuts, sugar and vinegar. Serve immediately.

1 Sandwich:

Calories 360
(Calories from Fat 80)
Fat 9g
Saturated Fat 3g
(8% of Calories from Saturated Fat)
Trans Fat 0g
Cholesterol 65mg
Omega-3 0g
Sodium 510mg

Exchanges:
2 1/2 Starch, 3 Lean Meat

1 Carbohydrate Choice

Ginger-Orange Bars

PREP: 25 min BAKE: 20 min COOL: 30 min
48 bars

Ingredients
1/2 cup butter, softened
1/2 cup whole wheat flour
1 1/2 cups all-purpose flour
1 teaspoon baking soda
1/4 teaspoon ground ginger
2 teaspoons grated orange peel

1/2 cup sugar
1 egg
1/2 cup molasses
2/3 cup buttermilk
Orange Frosting
  (below)

1 Serving:

Calories 110
(Calories from Fat 45)
Fat 5g
Saturated Fat 3g
(25% of Calories from
Saturated Fat)
Trans Fat 0g
Cholesterol 15mg
Omega-3 0g
Sodium 120mg

Exchanges:
1 Starch, 1/2 Fat

1 Heat oven to 350°. Spray jelly roll pan,
15 1/2 x 10 1/2 x 1 inch, with cooking spray.

2 Beat sugar and butter in large bowl with electric mixer on
medium speed until light and fluffy. Beat in molasses and egg.

3 Mix all-purpose flour, whole wheat flour, baking soda and
ginger in small bowl; add to sugar mixture alternately with
buttermilk, beating on low speed until blended. Stir in orange
peel. Spread in pan.

4 Bake 15 to 20 minutes or until toothpick inserted in center
comes out clean. Cool completely, about 30 minutes.

5 Meanwhile, make Orange Frosting. Spread frosting over
cooled bars. For bars, cut into 8 rows by 6 rows.

Orange Frosting
2 cups powdered sugar
1 tablespoon butter, softened
1/2 teaspoon grated orange peel
2 to 4 tablespoons orange juice

Mix all frosting ingredients in small bowl, adding enough orange
juice for desired spreading consistency; beat until smooth.

1 Carbohydrate Choice

Orchard Date-Apricot Bars

PREP: 20 min BAKE: 30 min COOL: 1 hr
36 bars

Ingredients

1 cup packed brown sugar
3/4 cup canola or soybean oil
3/4 cup all-purpose flour
1 cup plus 2 tablespoons ground
  flaxseed or flaxseed meal

1/2 teaspoon baking soda
1 teaspoon salt
1 1/2 cups quick-cooking oats

1   Make Date-Apricot Filling; cool. Heat oven to 400°. Spray rectangular pan, 13 x 9 x 2 inches, with cooking spray.

2   Mix brown sugar and oil in large bowl. Stir in remaining ingredients; mixture will be moist and crumbly. Press half of the crumb mixture evenly in bottom of pan. Spread with Date-Apricot Filling. Top with remaining crumb mixture; press lightly.

3   Bake 25 to 30 minutes or until lightly browned. Cool in pan on wire rack about 1 hour. For bars, cut into 6 rows by 6 rows.

Date-Apricot Filling

1 1/4 cups dates (8 ounces pitted)
1 1/2 cups dried apricots, cut up (8 ounces)
1/2 cup sugar
1 1/2 cups water

Mix all ingredients in a saucepan until well blended. Cook over medium-low heat, stirring constantly, until thickened, about 10 minutes.

1 Cookie:

Calories 155
(Calories from Fat 55)
Fat 6g
Saturated Fat 0g
(3% of Calories from Saturated Fat)
Trans Fat 0g
Cholesterol 0mg
Omega-3 1g
Sodium 90mg

Exchanges:
1/2 Starch, 1 Other Carbohydrates, 1 Fat

1.5 Carbohydrate Choices

Harvest Skillet Supper

PREP: 10 min COOK: 25 min
4 servings

Ingredients
3/4 cup apple juice
2 tablespoons Dijon mustard
2 teaspoons cornstarch
1 apple, cut into 16 wedges
2 teaspoons canola or soybean oil
1 cup uncooked instant brown rice
2 teaspoons packed brown sugar
1/2 cup coarsely chopped green bell pepper
3/4-pound pork tenderloin, cut into 1/4-inch slices
2 medium sweet potatoes, peeled, cut into
  1/4-inch slices (2 cups) or 2 cups sliced carrots

1 1/4 cups water
Dash of salt
Dash of pepper

1 Serving:

Calories 380
(Calories from Fat 65)
Fat 7g
Saturated Fat 2g
(4% of Calories from
Saturated Fat)
Trans Fat 0g
Cholesterol 55mg
Omega-3 0g
Sodium 300mg

Exchanges:
2 1/2 Starch, 1 Fruit,
2 1/2 Lean Meat

1   Heat oil in 10-inch nonstick skillet over medium-high heat. Cook pork in hot oil 2 to 3 minutes, turning once, until brown on both sides. Remove pork from skillet; cover to keep warm. Drain drippings from skillet.

2   Mix apple juice, mustard, cornstarch, brown sugar, salt and pepper in small bowl. Add to skillet with sweet potatoes; reduce heat. Cover and cook 10 to 15 minutes, stirring occasionally, until sweet potatoes are crisp-tender.

3   While sweet potatoes are cooking, heat water to boiling in medium saucepan; stir in rice. Reduce heat to low; cover and simmer 10 minutes.

4   Stir bell pepper, apple and pork into sweet potato mixture. Cover and cook 5 minutes longer, stirring occasionally, until bell pepper is crisp-tender and pork is no longer pink in center. Serve over rice; garnish with chopped fresh parsley if desired.

3.5 Carbohydrate Choices

Parmesan–White Bean Dip

PREP: 15 min COOK: 10 min
14 servings (2 tablespoons and 1/2 cup vegetables each)

Ingredients
1 tablespoon canola or soybean oil
2 cloves garlic, finely chopped
2 teaspoons chopped fresh or 1 teaspoon dried rosemary leaves, crumbled
1 can (19 ounces) cannellini beans, rinsed and drained
1/4 to 1/3 cup chicken broth or white wine
2 tablespoons chopped fresh Italian parsley
1 cup shredded Parmesan cheese (4 ounces)
7 cups assorted cut-up fresh vegetables

1 Heat oil in heavy 2-quart saucepan over medium heat. Cook garlic and rosemary in oil 1 to 2 minutes, stirring constantly, until garlic is light golden. Remove from heat.

2 Add cannellini beans and broth to saucepan. Partially mash beans with potato masher. Stir in parsley. Heat over medium-low heat, stirring occasionally, until bean mixture is thoroughly heated. Stir in cheese until melted. Serve warm with vegetables.

1 Serving:

Calories 125
(Calories from Fat 35)
Fat 4g
Saturated Fat 2g
(13% of Calories from
Saturated Fat)
Trans Fat 0g
Cholesterol 5mg
Omega-3 0g
Sodium 190mg

Exchanges:
1/2 Starch, 1 Vegetable,
1/2 Medium-Fat Meat,
1/2 Fat

2.5 Carbohydrate Choices

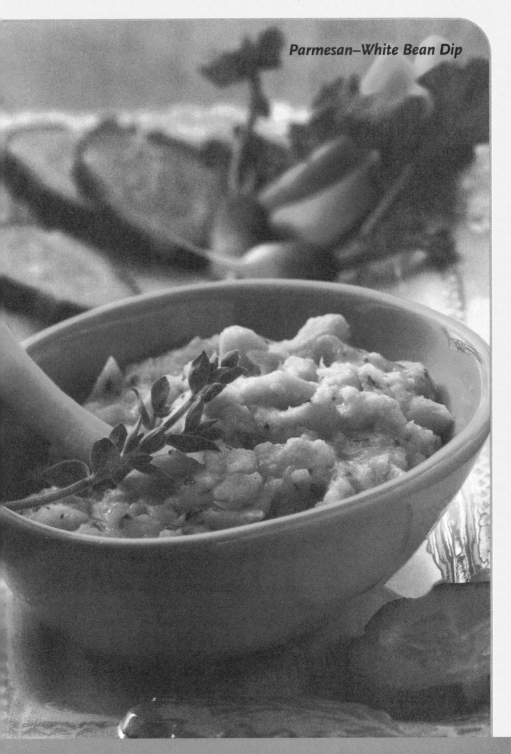

Parmesan–White Bean Dip

Peanut Butter–Raisin Breakfast Bars

PREP: 15 min STAND: 1 hr
12 bars

Ingredients
1/2 cup packed brown sugar
1/3 cup light corn syrup or honey
1/4 cup peanut butter
1/2 teaspoon ground cinnamon
4 cups Total® Raisin Bran cereal
1/2 cup chopped peanuts or sliced almonds

1   Butter square pan, 8 x 8 x 2 inches. Heat brown sugar and corn syrup just to boiling in 3-quart saucepan over medium heat, stirring frequently. Remove from heat; stir in peanut butter and cinnamon until smooth.

2   Stir in cereal and peanuts or almonds until evenly coated. Press firmly in pan. Let stand about 1 hour or until set. Cut into 4 rows by 3 rows. Store loosely covered at room temperature.

1 Bar:

Calories 200
(Calories from Fat 55)
Fat 6g
Saturated Fat 1g
(5% of Calories from Saturated Fat)
Trans Fat 0g
Cholesterol 0mg
Omega-3 0g
Sodium 170mg

Exchanges:
2 Starch, 1 Fat

2 Carbohydrate Choices

Oatmeal-Cranberry Muffins

PREP: 20 min BAKE: 25 min
12 muffins

Ingredients
1 cup buttermilk or sour milk
1 cup old-fashioned oats
3/4 cup packed brown sugar
1/3 cup canola or soybean oil
3/4 cup all-purpose flour
3/4 cup ground flaxseed or flaxseed meal
1 1/2 teaspoons baking powder
1 teaspoon salt
1 teaspoon ground cinnamon
1 cup fresh or frozen cranberries, chopped
1/4 cup fat-free cholesterol-free egg product,
    2 egg whites or 1 egg

1 Muffin:

Calories 215
(Calories from Fat 80)
Fat 9g
Saturated Fat 1g
(4% of Calories from
Saturated Fat)
Trans Fat 0g
Cholesterol 0mg
Omega-3 2g
Sodium 300mg

Exchanges:
2 Starch, 1 1/2 Fat

1   Heat oven to 400°. Pour buttermilk over oats in small bowl.
    Line 12 medium muffin cups, 2 1/2 x 1 1/4 inches, with paper
    baking cups.

2   Mix brown sugar, oil and egg product in large bowl. Stir in
    flour, flaxseed, baking powder, salt and cinnamon just until
    flour is moistened. Stir in oat mixture. Fold in cranberries.
    Divide batter evenly among muffin cups (about 3/4 full).

3   Bake 20 to 25 minutes or until toothpick inserted in center
    comes out clean. Immediately remove from pan. Serve warm.

2 Carbohydrate Choices

Parmesan Breaded Pork Chops

PREP: 10 min COOK: 18 min
4 servings

Ingredients
4 butterflied boneless pork loin chops, about 1/2 inch thick (about 1 pound)
1/3 cup Italian-style dry bread crumbs
2 tablespoons grated Parmesan cheese
1/4 cup fat-free cholesterol-free egg product or 2 egg whites
1 small green bell pepper, chopped (1/2 cup)
1 can (14 1/2 ounces) chunky tomatoes with olive oil, garlic and spices, undrained
1 can (8 ounces) tomato sauce

1   Trim fat from pork. Mix bread crumbs and cheese in shallow dish. Pour egg product into another shallow dish. Dip pork into egg product, then coat with crumb mixture.

2   Spray 12-inch nonstick skillet with cooking spray; heat over medium heat. Cook pork in skillet about 5 minutes, turning once, until brown on both sides.

3   Stir in remaining ingredients. Heat to boiling; reduce heat. Cover and simmer 10 to 12 minutes, stirring occasionally, until pork is no longer pink in center.

1 Serving:

Calories 290
(Calories from Fat 90)
Fat 10g
Saturated Fat 4g
(12% of Calories from Saturated Fat)
Trans Fat 0g
Cholesterol 70mg
Omega-3 0g
Sodium 860mg

Exchanges:
1 Vegetable, 1 Starch,
3 1/2 Lean Meat

1 Carbohydrate Choice

French Country-Style Peas

PREP: 5 min COOK: 5 min
4 servings

Ingredients
2 teaspoons canola or soybean oil
1/2 cup diced onion (1 medium)
1 cup sliced fresh mushrooms (about 2 1/2 ounces)
1 package (10 ounces) frozen peas and pearl onions
1/2 teaspoon salt
1/4 teaspoon white pepper
1 cup shredded romaine or Bibb lettuce
1 tablespoon minced fresh or 1 teaspoon dried tarragon or mint leaves,
   crushed

1   Heat oil in 10-inch nonstick skillet over
    medium heat. Cook onion in oil 1 minute,
    stirring occasionally. Stir in mushrooms
    and frozen vegetables; cook 3 minutes,
    stirring frequently. Stir in salt and pepper.

2   Stir in lettuce; cook 1 minute, stirring
    constantly, until lettuce is wilted. Sprinkle
    with tarragon.

1 Serving:

Calories 80
(Calories from Fat 25)
Fat 3g
Saturated Fat 0g
(3% of Calories from
Saturated Fat)
Trans Fat 0g
Cholesterol 0mg
Omega-3 0g
Sodium 330mg

Exchanges:
1/2 Fat, 2 Vegetable

1 Carbohydrate Choice

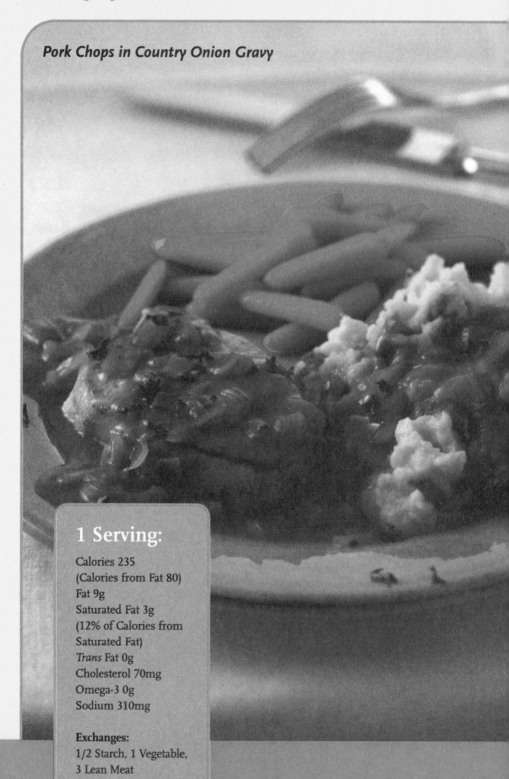

Pork Chops in Country Onion Gravy

1 Serving:

Calories 235
(Calories from Fat 80)
Fat 9g
Saturated Fat 3g
(12% of Calories from
Saturated Fat)
Trans Fat 0g
Cholesterol 70mg
Omega-3 0g
Sodium 310mg

Exchanges:
1/2 Starch, 1 Vegetable,
3 Lean Meat

Pork Chops in Country Onion Gravy

PREP: 10 min COOK: 24 min
4 servings

Ingredients
4 boneless pork loin chops (about 1 pound)
2 cups chopped onions
1 cup beef broth
1/8 teaspoon pepper
1/3 cup fat-free (skim) milk
2 tablespoons all-purpose flour

1 Generously spray 12-inch nonstick skillet with cooking spray; heat over medium-high heat. Cook pork chops in skillet about 6 minutes, turning once, until brown on both sides. Remove pork from skillet; cover to keep warm.

2 Reduce heat to medium. Add onions to skillet; cook 3 minutes. Stir in broth and pepper. Return pork to skillet; spoon onion mixture over pork. Cover tightly and simmer 12 minutes or until pork is no longer pink and meat thermometer inserted in center reads 160°.

3 Mix milk and flour in small bowl. Add to skillet; cook 2 to 3 minutes, stirring constantly, until thickened.

3 Carbohydrate Choices

Spanish Lamb and Couscous

PREP: 10 min COOK: 18 min
4 servings

Ingredients
4 lamb sirloin chops, 1/2 inch thick (about 2 pounds)
1 medium green bell pepper, chopped (1 cup)
1/4 cup chili sauce
1 can (14 1/2 ounces) diced tomatoes, undrained
1/2 teaspoon ground cumin
1/2 teaspoon dried marjoram leaves
1/4 teaspoon garlic powder
1/4 teaspoon salt
1/4 cup pitted ripe olives, cut in half
2 tablespoons chopped fresh parsley
2 cups hot cooked couscous

1 Spray 12-inch nonstick skillet with cooking spray; heat over medium heat. Cook lamb in skillet, turning once, until brown on both sides.

2 Stir in bell pepper, chili sauce, tomatoes, cumin, marjoram, garlic powder and salt; reduce heat to medium-low. Cover and simmer about 10 minutes or until lamb is light pink in center.

3 Stir in olives; sprinkle with parsley. Serve with couscous.

1 Serving:

Calories 320
(Calories from Fat 80)
Fat 9g
Saturated Fat 3g
(8% of Calories from
Saturated Fat)
Trans Fat 0g
Cholesterol 70mg
Omega-3 0g
Sodium 640mg

Exchanges:
2 Starch, 1 Vegetable,
1/2 Fat, 3 Very Lean Meat

2 Carbohydrate Choices

Glazed Baby Carrots and Cranberries with Pecans

PREP: 5 min COOK: 6 min
4 servings

Ingredients
1 package (10 ounces) frozen glazed sliced carrots in a
  pouch
3 tablespoons dried cranberries
2 tablespoons chopped pecans or walnuts

Cook carrots as directed on package. Stir in
cranberries and pecans.

1 Serving:

Calories 110
(Calories from Fat 45)
Fat 5g
Saturated Fat 1g
(6% of Calories from
Saturated Fat)
Trans Fat 0g
Cholesterol 0mg
Omega-3 0g
Sodium 230mg

Exchanges:
1 Fat, 1 Vegetable,
1/2 Other Carbohydrates

1 Carbohydrate Choice

Meal	Time	Blood Sugar	Food	Amount (cup, tablespoon, etc.)
Breakfast				
Snack				
Lunch				
Snack				
Dinner				
Snack				

See page 110 for an explanation of the Food Journal
Drinks: Please specify whether drinks are diet vs. regular
Condiments: Include items like sugar and cream in coffee or salt added to foods

Notes:

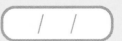

Meal	Time	Blood Sugar	Food	Amount (cup, tablespoon, etc.)
Breakfast				
Snack				
Lunch				
Snack				
Dinner				
Snack				

See page 110 for an explanation of the Food Journal
Drinks: Please specify whether drinks are diet vs. regular
Condiments: Include items like sugar and cream in coffee or salt added to foods

Notes:

Meal	Time	Blood Sugar	Food	Amount (cup, tablespoon, etc.)
Breakfast				
Snack				
Lunch				
Snack				
Dinner				
Snack				

See page 110 for an explanation of the Food Journal
Drinks: Please specify whether drinks are diet vs. regular
Condiments: Include items like sugar and cream in coffee or salt added to foods

Notes:

American College of Sports Medicine position stand. "The Recommended Quality and Quantity of Exercise for Developing and Maintaining Cardiorespiratory and Muscular Fitness in Healthy Adults." Medicine and Science in Sports and Exercise April 1990.

American Heart Association Consensus Panel Statement. "Preventing Heart Attack and Death in Patients With Coronary Disease." Circulation 1995; 2-4.

Burke, A.P., and A. Farb, G.T. Malcom, Y. Liang, J. Smialek, R. Virmani. "Coronary Risk Factors and Plaque Morphology in Men with Coronary Disease Who Died Suddenly." New England Journal of Medicine 1 May 1997: 1276-1282.

Cogswell, M.E. "Nicotine Withdrawal Symptoms." North Carolina Medical Journal 1 Jan. 1995: 40-45.

Danesh, J., J.G. Wheeler, G . Hirschfield, et al. "C-reactive protein and other circulation markers of inflammation in the prediction of coronary heart disease." New England Journal of Medicine 2004; 350:1387-1397.

Eckel, R.H. "Obesity in Heart Disease." Circulation 1997: 3248-3250.

Executive Summary of the Third Report of the National Cholesterol Education Program (NCEP) Expert Panel on Detection, Evaluation, and Treatment of High Blood Cholesterol in Adults (Adult Treatment Panel III). JAMA, May 16, 2001, Vol. 285, No. 19: 2486-2497.

Friedman, G.D., and A.L. Klatsky. "Is Alcohol Good for Your Health?" New England Journal of Medicine 16 Dec. 1993: 1882-1883.

Gellar, A. "Common Addictions." Clinical Symposia. Ciba-Geigy Corporation 1996.

Grundy, S.M., J.I. Cleeman, C.N.B. Merz et al. "Implications of recent clinical trials for the national cholesterol education program adult treatment panel III guidelines." Circulation 2004; 110:227-239.

Henningfield, J.D., and R.M. Keenan. "The Anatomy of Nicotine Addiction." Health Values March/April 1993: 12-19.

http://www.diabetes.org accessed on November 9, 2002

Joint National Committee. The Fifth Report of the Joint National Committee on Detection, Evaluation, and Treatment of High Blood Pressure. Bethesda (MD): National Institutes of Health, National Heart, Lung, and Blood Institute; 1993. NIH publication No. 93-1008.

Kannel, W.B., and R.B. D'Agostino, J.L. Cobb. "Effects of Weight on Cardiovascular Disease." American Journal of Clinical Nutrition March 1996: 419S-422S.

Kenney, W.L. et al. American College of Sports Medicine Guidelines for Exercise Testing and Prescription. 5th ed. Media, Pa.: Williams & Wilkins, 1995.

Koenig, W., H. Lowel, J. Baumert, and C. Mesisinger. "C-reactive protein modulates risk prediction based on the Framingham score. Implications for future risk assessment: results from a large cohort study in Southern Germany." Circulation 2004; 109:1349-1353.

McCarron, D.A., and M.E. Reusser. "Body Weight and Blood Pressure Regulation." American Journal of Clinical Nutrition March 1996: 423S-425S.

Pearson, T.A.,G.A. Mensah, R.W. Aleander, et al. "Markers of inflammation and cardiovascular disease. Application to clinical and public health practice." Circulation 2003; 107:499-511.

Peterson, J.A., and C.X. Bryant, The Fitness Handbook; 2nd edition, St. Louis: Wellness Bookshelf, 1995.

Peterson, T.A., G.A. Mensah, and R.W. Alexander et al. "Markers of inflammation and cardiovascular disease. Application to clinical and public health practice." Circulation 2003; 107:499-511.

Ridker, P.M. "Clinical application of C-reactive protein for cardiovascular disease detection and prevention." Circulation 2003; 107: 363-369.

Ridker, P.M., J.E. Buring, N.R. Cook, and N. Rifai. "C-reactive protein, the metabolic syndrome and risk of incident cardiovascular events: an 8-year follow-up of 14,719 initially healthy American women." Circulation 2003; 107;391-397.

Ridker, P.M., N. Rifai, and L. Rose, et al. "Comparison of C-reactive protein and low-density lipoprotein cholesterol levels in the prediction of first cardiovascular events." New England Journal of Medicine 2002; 347:1557-1565.

Ryan, T.J., and J.L. Anderson, E.M. Autman, et al. "ACC/AHA Guidelines for the Management of Patients with Acute Myocardial Infarction: A Report of the American College of Cardiology/American Heart Association Task Force on Practice Guidelines (Committee on Management of Acute Myocardial Infarction)." Journal of the American College of Cardiology 1 Nov. 1996: 1328-1428.

St. Jeor, S.T., and K.D. Brownell, R.L. Atkinson, C. Bouchard, et al. "Obesity Workshop III." Circulation 1996: 1391-1396.

Superko, H.R. "The Most Common Cause of Coronary Heart Disease can be Successfully Treated by the Least Expensive Therapy — Exercise." Certified News 1998: 1-5.

United States Surgeon General. Department of Health and Human Services. The Health Consequences of Smoking. Nicotine Addiction. Washington, D.C.: U.S. Department of Health and Human Services, 1988.

United States Surgeon General on his priorities at http://www.osophs.dhhs.gov/myjob/priorities.htm accessed November 1999.

Voors, A.A., et al. "Smoking and Cardiac Events After Venous Coronary Bypass Surgery." Circulation Jan 1, 1995: 42-47.

White H.D., and J.J. Van de Werf. "Thrombolysis for Acute Myocardial Infarction." Circulation 28 April 1998: 1632-1646.

Yeh, E.T.H., and J.T. Willerson. "Coming of age of C-reactive protein: using inflammation markers in cardiology." Circulation 2003; 107:370-372.

Date	BP	TC	Trig	LDL	HDL	Glucose	A1c	Comments
	—							
	—							
	—							
	—							
	—							
	—							
	—							
	—							
	—							
	—							
	—							
	—							
	—							

Target Values:

Blood Pressure (BP) . Less than 130/80 mm Hg
Before Meal Glucose . 80 mg/dL to 120 mg/dL
A1C . . . . Less than 7%

Total Cholesterol (TC) . . Less than 200mg/dL
Triglycerides (Trig) . . . . . Less than 150 mg/dL
LDL-Cholesterol . . . . Less than 70 mg/dL
HDL-Cholesterol . . . . . . Greater than 40 mg/dL
for men and greater than
50 mg/dL for women